THE MANY FACES OF ADHD

The Breakthrough Guide to Understanding Your Brain, Identifying Your Subtype, and Finding the Treatment That Finally Works

DR DONA BISWAS
MBBS, MD (PSYCHIATRY), FRANZP, BCN
DR VIVEK SHARMA
MBBS, MD (PSYCHIATRY), BCN, QEEG-D

The Many Faces of ADHD

For more information, address: quantumpsychiatrist@gmail.com

FIRST EDITION

ISBN-13: 978-0-6488651-2-4

Table of Contents

PART THREE

Disclaimer

This book is written for educational and informational purposes only. It is not intended as medical advice, clinical diagnosis, or a substitute for assessment and treatment by a qualified healthcare professional. Nothing here should be taken as a recommendation to begin, change, or discontinue any medication, supplement, or treatment without first consulting a qualified medical practitioner familiar with your individual circumstances.

The ADHD subtype framework described in Part Two is derived primarily from functional neuroimaging (SPECT) and quantitative EEG (QEEG) research, and draws substantially on the work of Daniel G. Amen MD and others. Readers should be aware that this subtype model, while clinically well-established within the neuroimaging traditions, is not currently standard diagnostic nomenclature in mainstream psychiatry. The DSM-5 recognises three clinical presentations of ADHD and does not incorporate neuroimaging-based subtyping as part of the formal diagnostic process. Similarly, the supplement protocols and functional testing approaches in Part Three reflect integrative psychiatry frameworks that, while evidence-informed, are not universally endorsed by conventional psychiatric guidelines.

The composite characters throughout this book — Liam, Priya, Oliver, Zara, Daniel, Maya, and Amir — are fictional composites drawn from broad clinical experience and do not represent any specific individual. The authors and publisher have made every effort to ensure accuracy at the time of publication, but medicine is a rapidly evolving field and readers are encouraged to consult current literature and qualified practitioners accordingly. The authors and publisher disclaim responsibility for any adverse outcomes arising from application of the information contained herein.

Dedication

To our parents, and to our Spiritual Master — without whom neither we nor this work would have been possible.

Acknowledgements

This book would not exist without the patients who have trusted us with their brains, their stories, and their struggles over many years of clinical practice. It is their courage in seeking answers beyond the standard prescription — and their willingness to look at their neurobiology with curiosity rather than resignation — that has shaped every page of this work. We are also deeply grateful to the researchers, clinicians, and scientists whose life's work underpins the integrative framework described here: Daniel Amen, James Greenblatt, Joel Lubar, Jay Gunkelman, John Johnstone, Russell Barkley, and the many others whose dedication to understanding the brain behind the diagnosis has expanded what psychiatric care can offer.

We are grateful to our families for their patience, encouragement, and graceful tolerance of the particular variety of preoccupation that accompanies writing a book of this scope. We would also like to acknowledge the broader community of integrative practitioners, neurofeedback clinicians, and functional medicine researchers who are quietly, persistently building a better model of care — often outside the mainstream, and rarely with the recognition they deserve. Your work matters. And to each other: this book is the product of a collaboration built on shared conviction, mutual respect, and the occasional very long conversation about QEEG patterns at inconvenient hours. We would not have it any other way.

~ Dr. Dona Biswas and Dr. Vivek Sharma

Introduction
The Brain Is Not a Checklist

Here is a small confession.

One of the authors of this book spent the better part of three years quietly convinced he had ADHD. The evidence was, on reflection, fairly compelling: the perpetually cluttered desk, the half-read books stacked in optimistic towers around the office, the startling number of projects that were almost finished. The capacity to spend four hours reading about something that interested him and approximately eleven minutes on something that didn't. The keys. Always, inexplicably, the keys.

So he did what any responsible psychiatrist would do: he assessed himself using exactly the same clinical tools he used with patients. He worked through a structured interview, completed standardised rating scales, and reviewed the DSM-5 criteria with what he hoped was appropriate objectivity. He scored well above the diagnostic threshold for combined-type ADHD. The checklist said: yes.

And then he looked at his own brain.

His QEEG — the quantitative electroencephalogram, a map of the brain's electrical activity recorded through sensors on the scalp

— told a substantially different story. Not the high-theta, low-beta signature that characterises classic ADHD, the pattern of cortical underactivation that stimulant medications are designed to address. Instead, his brain showed excessive high-frequency activity across the frontal lobes: the unmistakable fingerprint of a system running too fast, too hot, too close to the edge of exhaustion for too long. Not an underactivated brain. An overactivated one. Not ADHD. Burnout — with attentional consequences that looked, from the outside, identical to ADHD but required treatment that was, in important respects, opposite in direction.

Stimulant medication would have made things worse. Significantly worse.

This book was born from that moment — and from the hundred clinical encounters that surrounded it, in which patients arrived carrying a diagnosis that was descriptively accurate and aetiologically uninformative, having received treatments selected by category rather than by neurobiology. Some of them were helped. Many were not. All of them deserved better.

The Most Talked-About Diagnosis Nobody Fully Understands

ADHD — Attention Deficit Hyperactivity Disorder — is, depending on who you ask, either the most underdiagnosed condition of the modern age or the most over-medicated one. Both positions are held simultaneously, by intelligent and well-intentioned people, often in the same journal issue. This is not because the researchers involved are confused. It is because both positions contain genuine truth, and the tension between them reflects something important about the nature of the diagnosis itself.

Between five and ten per cent of the global population meets formal diagnostic criteria for ADHD. Millions more live with symptoms that fall just below the clinical threshold — close enough to cause real and lasting difficulty, not quite close enough to cross the line on a rating scale. The condition is associated with higher rates of academic failure, accidents, unemployment, substance misuse, relationship breakdown, and incarceration. It costs economies billions in lost productivity and untreated mental health consequences. It is real, it is widespread, and it matters enormously.

And yet, for all its prevalence, ADHD remains profoundly misunderstood — by the general public, by many clinicians, and arguably by the diagnostic systems we use to define it. The problem is not that ADHD doesn't exist. It does. The problem is that what we call ADHD almost certainly is not one thing. It is a family of related conditions — different brains, wired differently, producing similar but not identical difficulties — all handed the same label and, far too often, the same prescription.

What This Book Is About

This is a book about brains, not behaviours. Or more precisely: it is a book about why you cannot understand behaviour until you understand the brain producing it.

Modern psychiatric diagnosis is, at its core, behavioural. Clinicians observe what people do — or fail to do — and match those patterns against criteria in a diagnostic manual. This process has genuine value: it creates a shared clinical language, guides research, and helps identify people who need support. But behaviours are the last thing to emerge from a cascade of biological events. By the time a child is bouncing off the walls of a classroom, or an adult is staring at an unstarted task at midnight for the third consecutive evening, dozens of upstream processes — genetic, neurochemical, electrophysiological, nutritional — have already shaped what we are seeing.

This book goes upstream.

We draw on integrative psychiatry — a model of care that uses the full toolkit of neuroscience alongside rigorous evidence-based complementary approaches — and on the insights made available by quantitative electroencephalography (QEEG) and neurofeedback. We also draw on decades of combined clinical experience working with hundreds of individuals who were struggling with attention, focus, impulse control, and cognitive regulation. Some of them had ADHD. Many had conditions that looked like ADHD but weren't. Some had both. All of them deserved more than a fifteen-minute assessment and a repeat prescription.

The work of clinicians who pioneered brain-imaging approaches to attention disorders — especially Daniel Amen's SPECT imaging research provides essential foundation. The seven subtypes which we talk about are his terminology. We also draw on the integrative framework of psychiatrists like James Greenblatt. We build on these understandings, and where our own clinical and research experience warrants it, we extend it.

The Seven People You Are About to Meet

Research is most compelling when it lives inside a human being.

Throughout this book, seven people will carry the ideas we are exploring. They are composites, drawn from years of clinical practice — real in every way that matters. Each carries a different expression of what we call ADHD. Each has a different brain. Each will require a different approach. They will appear at the opening of each chapter, and surface again wherever their particular story illuminates what we are discussing.

> ***LIAM, 9 — Classic ADHD / Combined Type:*** *The boy who has never, in his entire conscious life, sat still without an ulterior motive. His classroom is his nemesis; the playground, his kingdom. He has been sent out of class eleven times this term. He is not sorry. He would do it again. His teacher's latest note home reads: 'Liam is bright, energetic, and genuinely exhausting.' His parents are beginning to agree with all three parts of that sentence, in descending order of comfort.*
>
> ***PRIYA, 11 — Inattentive Type:*** *Quiet, polite, and perpetually somewhere else. She doesn't cause trouble; she drifts. Her teachers call her 'a little dreamy.' Her parents assume she's shy. Nobody suspects that she has been missing half of every lesson since Year Three, not because she is inattentive in any visible sense, but because she is invisible — present in body, absent in mind, in ways that a rating scale completed by relieved teachers will never catch.*
>
> ***OLIVER, 34 — Overfocused Type:*** *Won every academic prize available and cannot understand why his marriage, his team, and his inbox are quietly falling apart. He can spend six unbroken hours on a problem that fascinates him. He cannot spend twenty minutes on one that doesn't. When he is interrupted mid-task, something in him goes rigid with fury before he can suppress it. He does not think he has ADHD. He thinks ADHD is for children who can't sit still. He is wrong, and it is costing him everything.*
>
> ***ZARA, 28 — Ring of Fire Type:*** *Everything is too loud. The fluorescent lights in the waiting room were genuinely painful. She has been misdiagnosed with bipolar disorder twice, and her second psychiatrist called her 'treatment resistant,' which is doctor for 'we've run out of ideas.' She is neither bipolar nor resistant. She is a person whose brain runs at a frequency*

that the diagnostic manual doesn't have a name for yet. She is brilliant, combustible, and very, very tired.

DANIEL, 42 — Temporal Lobe Type: *Daniel has been made redundant three times, and each time it has genuinely surprised him. Warning signs delivered in conversation simply don't reach him the way they should — spoken words arrive, seem to register, and dissolve before they can be acted on. He can recall, with aching vividness, an argument from 2009. He cannot recall what was discussed in Tuesday's meeting. He has a short fuse that bewilders him — not a constant combustibility, but sudden storms that arrive from nowhere, pass quickly, and leave him wondering what on earth just happened. He has been meaning to get help for years. The thought keeps losing its thread.*

MAYA, 38 — Limbic / Mood-Dysregulated Type: *Brilliant at her job, when she can get out of her own way. Her manager said 'good work' last week instead of 'excellent work' and she spent the following three hours constructing a detailed theory of imminent dismissal. She has been told she is 'too sensitive' her whole life. She has started to suspect the problem is not her sensitivity but the absence of anyone who has ever looked at what is actually happening in her brain.*

AMIR, 32 — Anxious Type: *Polished and professional, quiet and immaculate. Smart enough to hold things together; anxious enough to never feel safe. He avoids conflict, second-guesses every decision, and lies awake at 3 a.m. replaying conversations from 2018. He has seventeen browser tabs open about updating his CV. He will open seventeen more. Every time he has plucked the courage to ask for help, the result has been disappointing.*

These seven people share a diagnosis. They do not share a brain. By the time this book is finished, the distinction will feel not just intellectually important but clinically urgent.

A Map of What Lies Ahead

Part One lays the foundations. We examine how ADHD came to be defined, what the current diagnostic criteria capture and what they miss, why the controversies surrounding this condition are more substantive than clinical guidelines typically acknowledge, the neuroscience of how attention is regulated and how it fails, and the evidence on long-term treatment that somehow manages not to appear in most clinical conversations.

Part Two zooms in. We explore the tools that allow us to see the brain rather than just observe the behaviour: continuous performance tests and what they measure, quantitative EEG and the phenotypic framework that moves assessment beyond DSM categories, and — in individual chapters — each of the seven major neurobiological ADHD subtypes. For each, we examine the QEEG signature, the SPECT imaging correlates, the neurochemical profile, and the specific implications for medication, supplements, and neurofeedback.

Part Three turns to treatment. We examine the problems with current medications for long-term use, with honesty about what the evidence actually shows. We then offer a structured integrative approach: functional testing, dietary strategies, lifestyle foundations, targeted supplementation, and medication when appropriate — all calibrated to the specific brain rather than the general label.

Let us begin where ADHD actually begins: not in a diagnostic manual, but in the longer, stranger, and considerably more illuminating story of how the diagnosis arrived, and what came before it.

PART ONE

The Label Is Not the Brain

The five chapters that follow are, in one sense, a preparation for everything that comes after. But they are also worth reading carefully on their own terms — because understanding what ADHD is, where it came from, what the research actually shows, and what the diagnostic process systematically misses is not background material. It is the substance of the clinical problem this book is trying to solve.

We will meet Liam, Priya, Oliver, Zara, Daniel, Maya and Amir at the opening of each chapter — always a little older, always revealing a little more. We will examine the history of a diagnosis that has been reshaped more times than most people realise, the scientific foundations that are stronger than critics suggest and weaker than proponents admit, and the evidence on long-term outcomes that has somehow remained much better known to researchers than to patients.

By the end of Part One, we hope you will understand why looking at the label is not enough — and why looking at the brain is not optional.

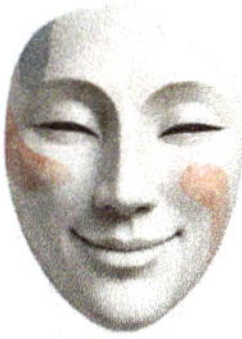

Chapter One

Through the Mirrors of Time

A history of ADHD — and the drug that got there first

> ***LIAM — Age 9:*** *'He's bright, but he just can't behave,' his teacher writes in the Year Four report. 'Constantly out of his seat. Distracts other children. Wonderful imagination, if only we could get him to use it.' His parents take him to the GP. The GP refers him for ADHD assessment. The waiting list is eight months. In the meantime, Liam gets three more detentions, successfully removes the arm from a waiting room chair, and teaches himself to skateboard from YouTube videos he watches instead of doing homework. He is, by any measure, thriving. The system around him is not.*

> ***PRIYA — Age 11:*** *Her report says: 'A pleasure to have in class. Could try harder.' Nobody has noticed that Priya has been trying, desperately and privately, every single day — and still arriving home unable to recall what was on the board that morning. She rewrites her notes three times. She reads the chapter twice. She sits at the front. None of it helps. She is not a problem child. She is invisible. And invisible children wait a very long time for help.*

Here is something most people do not know about ADHD: the medication came first.

The drugs prescribed to millions of children and adults every morning — amphetamine salts, methylphenidate, and their various extended-release incarnations — were not developed in response to ADHD research. They were not designed with attentional neuroscience in mind. They arrived decades before the diagnosis existed, were prescribed initially for entirely different conditions, and the discovery that they affected children's behaviour and focus was, in the most literal sense, accidental. A side observation. A pleasant surprise that medicine then spent the next eighty years building an industry around.

This is not a minor footnote in the history of the condition. It is the foundational fact about ADHD treatment, and it shapes — in ways both obvious and subtle — the clinical landscape that patients and practitioners navigate today.

To understand how we arrived at a world where an eleven-minute appointment and a rating scale completed by a teacher can determine whether a seven-year-old receives a Schedule II controlled substance, we need to go back. Much further back than most people realise.

The Oldest Complaint in the World

Descriptions of what we now call ADHD predate the discipline of psychiatry by a very considerable margin. Hippocrates — yes, that Hippocrates, the one with the oath and the barely-surviving diet recommendations — described, around 460 BC, individuals whose attention shifted too rapidly with external stimuli, who perceived everything with unusual acuity and retained nothing for long. He attributed the condition, as he attributed most things, to an excess of fire in the blood. His treatment: green vegetables, barley, water, sports, and 'a fish diet.' Remarkably, three of these recommendations have since accumulated credible evidence, and the fish component has turned out to be particularly well-founded. Hippocrates, in this as in much else, was ahead of his time.

In 1798, the Scottish physician Sir Alexander Crichton published a book with the gloriously Victorian title *An Inquiry into the Nature and Origin of Mental Derangement* — a title that has the advantage of complete honesty about the state of the field at the time, and would still be defensible today. In it, Crichton described patients with what he called 'the disease of attention': an inability to fix the mind on any object for any length of time, combined with extraordinary responsiveness to external stimuli. These were not unintelligent people, he was at pains to note. Their capacity for reason was intact. Something in the regulatory machinery of attention itself was simply not working as expected.

John Locke, writing a century before Crichton, made similar observations about students who could not sustain concentration during study. Various physicians across the intervening centuries had noted the phenomenon in their case reports without having any particular framework for it. The behaviours, in other words, were always there. What was missing was the consistent clinical language, the diagnostic category, and — crucially — any workable treatment.

Still's Children — When Medicine Got Involved

The first genuinely systematic clinical account is usually attributed to the British paediatrician Sir George Frederick Still, who in 1902 delivered three lectures to the Royal College of Physicians describing a series of children who showed what he called 'an abnormal defect of moral control.' The language is jarring to modern ears — 'moral control' sounds like a Victorian Sunday school lesson — but Still's clinical observations were acute. These children were restless, impulsive, easily distracted, and unable to regulate their behaviour in ways appropriate to their age, despite, he noted carefully, having entirely normal intelligence. They weren't unintelligent. They weren't wilfully disobedient. Something in their regulatory system wasn't working as it should.

Still's description has another quality worth noting: the disproportionate representation of boys in his case series. Many of his twenty cases were male. The gender imbalance in ADHD identification — which persists to this day, with girls like Priya remaining dramatically and consequentially underdiagnosed — begins here, in the founding clinical observations, written into the literature from its very first page.

Three decades later, in 1932, the German physicians Franz Kramer and Hans Pollnow described children with extreme motor restlessness and impulsivity, calling the condition 'hyperkinetic disease of infancy.' The behaviours were being named. They were being categorised and argued over in medical journals. But they still lacked any biological explanation — or any treatment. That was about to change, in a way nobody had quite anticipated.

The Drug That Arrived Before the Diagnosis

Before we examine how amphetamine found its way to children, it is worth pausing on a page from history that quietly dismantles one of the most persistent myths in ADHD pharmacology: that stimulant medications work specifically and uniquely in ADHD brains, those who don't have ADHD react differently, and that their effectiveness in the ADHD population constitutes evidence of an underlying neurological deficit. The history that follows suggests otherwise.

In 1929, a biochemist named Gordon Alles was searching for a cheaper substitute for ephedrine — at the time expensive and difficult to obtain — to treat asthma and nasal congestion. He synthesised a compound he called amphetamine. While testing it on himself, which was entirely standard pharmacological practice at the time and speaks to a certain admirable willingness to be one's own experimental subject, he noticed that his mood lifted, his energy surged considerably, and his focus sharpened. He filed a patent. Smith, Kline and French bought it.

By 1933, Smith, Kline and French were selling an amphetamine inhaler under the name Benzedrine — marketed for nasal congestion, available over the counter, stocked in every pharmacy. By the late 1930s, tablets were being promoted for a remarkable range of indications: narcolepsy, mild depression, 'fatigue,' and the loosely defined condition that physicians of the era called 'neurotic exhaustion.' The American Medical Association had approved amphetamine for twelve separate conditions by 1937. Psychiatrists enthusiastically adopted it as what many considered the first pharmacological antidepressant. SKF-funded Harvard psychiatrist Abraham Myerson theorised that amphetamine 'adjusted hormonal balance' in the central nervous system, promoting activity and extraversion. The precise mechanism was unclear. The commercial enthusiasm was not.

The connection to children came the same year. Charles Bradley, a psychiatrist working at a residential school for children with neurological and behavioural difficulties in Providence, Rhode Island, began administering Benzedrine to thirty children in his care. He had intended it primarily to treat headaches caused by the diagnostic procedures he was performing. What he observed instead was something entirely unexpected: more than half of the children showed dramatic improvements in academic performance, mood, and behaviour. Teachers reported that children who had previously struggled were suddenly completing their work correctly and promptly. The staff began calling Benzedrine 'the arithmetic pill.'

Bradley published his findings in the American Journal of Psychiatry in 1937. The medical establishment received them with polite interest — and then largely ignored them for nearly two decades. The world was not yet ready for the idea of medicating children's behaviour. The diagnosis that would eventually justify this approach didn't exist yet. And the pharmaceutical machinery that would ultimately industrialise Bradley's observation was still being assembled. The seed, however, had been planted.

The First Epidemic — The One Nobody Talks About

During the 1940s and 1950s, amphetamine use expanded far beyond its original medical indications, and began to reveal what uninhibited availability of a stimulant compound looks like at a population level.

Students used it to study longer. Workers used it to increase output. Writers and artists used it through the night. The Second World War accelerated consumption dramatically: Britain, Germany, the United States, and Japan all distributed amphetamines to military personnel. The RAF issued Benzedrine to bomber crews for long missions. The Wehrmacht distributed Pervitin — methamphetamine — so liberally that German soldiers called it 'tank chocolate.' Millions of servicemen encountered the drug during the war years, many for the first time.

The postwar civilian market told a similar story. By the early 1960s, the United States alone was producing enough amphetamine for every American to receive dozens of doses annually. Historian Nicolas Rasmussen's landmark 2008 paper in the American Journal of Public Health documented this period in detail, characterising it as America's 'first amphetamine epidemic' — one that was primarily iatrogenic, generated not by clandestine drug markets but by the routine commercial activities of pharmaceutical companies and the prescribing practices of physicians who trusted their promotional materials (Rasmussen, 2008). Approximately 85% of the amphetamine prescriptions at the epidemic's peak were written for women aged 36 to 45, primarily for depression and weight management — a demographic detail that sits in uncomfortable proximity to the modern anxiety about overprescribing for ADHD.

By the late 1960s, the consequences of unrestricted prescribing had become impossible to ignore. Clinicians documented amphetamine psychosis — paranoid, hallucinatory, indistinguishable from acute schizophrenia — in patients who had begun with entirely ordinary prescriptions. Evidence of dependence, tolerance, and diversion accumulated. Public concern about stimulant abuse mounted. In 1971, the Controlled Substances Act placed amphetamine on Schedule II, the same classification it carries today — acknowledging its abuse potential while preserving its medical use.

Rasmussen's paper contained a finding that deserves to be read by every prescribing clinician in the field: current prescribed stimulant consumption in the United States has returned, in absolute terms, to roughly the same levels as at the epidemic's peak in 1969 — and it has done so not in the absence of regulation, but in spite of it. The Schedule II classification that ended the first epidemic remains in place. The prescriptions are being written anyway.

How ADHD Got Its Name — The Classification Wars

While stimulant use was following its own trajectory, psychiatric diagnostic frameworks were evolving in parallel — and eventually the two tracks converged, with consequences that shape clinical practice to this day.

The first edition of the Diagnostic and Statistical Manual of Mental Disorders, published in 1952, did not contain ADHD. What it contained, under the category of 'Minimal Brain Damage,' was a label that had the virtue of descriptive honesty and the disadvantage of being simultaneously stigmatising and largely unsupported by neurological evidence. Minimal brain damage implied something was wrong with the brain. The evidence that anything was structurally wrong was thin. The label stuck anyway.

DSM-II in 1968 replaced this with 'Hyperkinetic Reaction of Childhood' — acknowledging the motor component while making no claims about underlying neurobiology. Progress, of a kind.

The genuine watershed came with DSM-III in 1980, which introduced 'Attention Deficit Disorder' — with or without hyperactivity. This was a meaningful scientific advance. For the first time, inattention was formally recognised as a core feature that could exist without hyperactivity, opening the diagnostic door for the quieter, dreamier, non-disruptive presentations that would eventually become the Predominantly Inattentive type. It meant that children like Priya — causing no trouble, noticed by nobody, simply not learning — could, theoretically, be identified.

In practice, they mostly weren't. But theoretically, the door was open.

DSM-III-R in 1987 reorganised the criteria, and by DSM-IV in 1994 the framework we still recognise had arrived: ADHD with three presentations — Combined, Predominantly Inattentive, and Predominantly Hyperactive-Impulsive. DSM-5, published in 2013, made several significant adjustments: it raised the symptom onset age from seven to twelve (making adult diagnosis more accessible), reduced the symptom threshold for adults from six to five criteria, and replaced 'subtypes' with 'presentations,' acknowledging that individuals might shift between them over time. The terminology changed. The underlying biology remained as poorly captured as it had ever been.

Each revision of the diagnostic criteria was accompanied by a measurable expansion of the diagnosable population. Each expansion was accompanied by an increase in prescribing. This is not necessarily sinister — improved recognition of a genuinely impairing condition is a legitimate reason for increased diagnosis. But when diagnostic criteria expand reliably in directions that increase the commercially available market for existing medications, the epistemic vigilance required of clinicians and policymakers alike is correspondingly higher.

The Numbers — And What They Do and Don't Tell Us

In the United States, ADHD diagnoses in children rose from approximately 7.8% in 2003 to 11.3% by 2016. In some Southern states, rates exceed 14%. Adult ADHD diagnoses more than doubled between 2007 and 2016. Global prevalence estimates for adult ADHD hover around 2.5–5%, though methodological differences between studies complicate direct comparison.

These numbers reflect multiple overlapping realities. Genuine improvements in recognition — particularly of inattentive presentations in girls and women who were previously systematically invisible to criteria built around hyperactive boys. Reduced stigma enabling more people to seek assessment. Broader diagnostic criteria capturing previously subthreshold presentations. Increased public awareness, driven in part by the extraordinary reach of social media communities. And, in some markets, commercial pressures from an industry whose revenues depend on an expanding patient pool — a factor that receives less acknowledgement in clinical literature than in public health research.

What these numbers cannot tell us — and this is the central limitation — is whether the individuals receiving diagnoses share the same underlying neurobiology, or whether the ADHD umbrella covers an increasingly heterogeneous collection of brain states that happen to produce similar behavioural presentations. The evidence strongly suggests the latter. Understanding why that matters is what the rest of this book is about.

What History Actually Teaches Us

The history of ADHD is not a straightforward story of scientific progress — of ignorance yielding steadily to enlightenment, of better evidence producing better outcomes. It is a story of genuine clinical observations being filtered through changing social values, commercial interests, evolving diagnostic fashions, and the institutional pressures of a profession whose categorical tools have consistently outrun its biological understanding.

Three things emerge from this history that matter for everything that follows.

The first is that the medication arrived before the diagnosis and has barely changed since. The core pharmacological treatment for ADHD in 2026 is functionally the same class of compound Charles Bradley administered to children in 1937. Nearly ninety years of neuroscientific progress, and the first-line response remains substantially unaltered. Either the molecule is remarkably well-suited to the problem — which is true for some presentations — or we have not looked hard enough for alternatives. This book argues for the latter, and provides evidence for why looking harder is both warranted and clinically productive.

The second is that the diagnosis has always been descriptive, never explanatory. 'ADHD' describes a cluster of behaviours that clinicians have agreed, through committee votes and iterative revision, to call a disorder. It does not explain what is causing those behaviours in any individual brain. This distinction — between description and explanation — is not semantic. It determines whether treatment is targeted or generic, whether it addresses causes or suppresses symptoms, and whether it has any realistic prospect of producing lasting change.

The third is that the gap between what the evidence shows and what the clinical and commercial system disseminates has been, at times, substantial. As we will see in later chapters, the follow-up data from the most important treatment study ever conducted on ADHD received a fraction of the attention that the original headline findings generated. The study was the same. The results were different. The dissemination was not equal.

In the next chapter, we turn to the diagnosis itself — not in the polemical terms of the culture wars that have surrounded ADHD for thirty years, but in the precise clinical language of what the DSM requires, what the research supports, what it fails to capture, and why the symptoms that millions of people find most debilitating somehow never made it into the manual.

References — Chapter One

Crichton, A. (1798). An Inquiry into the Nature and Origin of Mental Derangement. London: T. Cadell and W. Davies.

Still, G.F. (1902). 'Some abnormal psychical conditions in children: the Goulstonian Lectures.' The Lancet, 159(4103), 1008–1012.

Bradley, C. (1937). 'The behavior of children receiving Benzedrine.' American Journal of Psychiatry, 94(3), 577–585.

Rasmussen, N. (2008). 'America's first amphetamine epidemic 1929–1971: a quantitative and qualitative retrospective.' American Journal of Public Health, 98(6), 974–985.

Barkley, R.A. (2015). Attention-Deficit Hyperactivity Disorder: A Handbook for Diagnosis and Treatment (4th ed.). New York: Guilford Press.

American Psychiatric Association. (2013). Diagnostic and Statistical Manual of Mental Disorders (5th ed.). Washington, DC: APA.

Faraone, S.V. et al. (2021). 'The World Federation of ADHD International Consensus Statement: 208 evidence-based conclusions about the disorder.' Neuroscience & Biobehavioral Reviews, 128, 789–818.

Conrad, P. (2007). The Medicalization of Society. Baltimore: Johns Hopkins University Press.

Berman, S.M., Kuczenski, R., McCracken, J.T. & London, E.D. (2009). 'Potential adverse effects of amphetamine treatment on brain and behavior: a review.' Molecular Psychiatry, 14(2), 123–142.

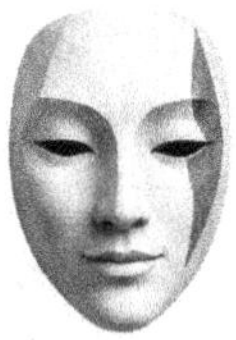

Chapter Two

What ADHD Is — And Isn't

The diagnosis, the debates, and the symptoms nobody put in the manual

> ***OLIVER — Age 16:*** *Every teacher loves Oliver. He sits at the front of every class, reads every book on every topic before he needs to, and produces work of a quality that generates sincere admiration and mild resentment in equal measure among his peers. Nobody notices that when Oliver is interrupted mid-task — when the bell rings, when dinner is called, when someone knocks — something in him goes rigid with fury that takes several seconds to suppress. Nobody notices because he suppresses it perfectly. The cost of this focus, paid entirely in private.*
>
> ***LIAM — Age 14, Five Years On:*** *Liam has been suspended three times this year. His school has suggested that perhaps 'a different educational environment might suit him better,' which is administrative euphemism for 'please take him somewhere else before he costs us any more.' His mother cries at the kitchen table. Liam himself claims not to be particularly bothered. He has found that skateboarding, petty shoplifting, and wiring up a basic electrical circuit all provide the intensity his brain is constantly seeking. One of these is significantly more socially acceptable than the others.*

Ask ten people to define ADHD and you will get eleven answers.

Ask ten psychiatrists, and you might get twelve — because several of them will offer a nuanced revision of their initial position before you have finished writing it down. This is not intellectual inconsistency. It is an honest response to a genuinely complicated question about a genuinely complicated condition.

ADHD is one of the most researched conditions in all of psychiatry, and one of the most contested. Not because the research is poor — much of it is excellent, rigorous, and illuminating. But because the question of what, precisely, we are measuring when we apply this diagnosis is difficult in ways that matter clinically, and difficult questions attract disagreement proportional to their clinical importance.

This chapter tries to give an honest account of what ADHD is, as formally defined; what the diagnostic criteria actually capture and what they systematically miss; why the debate about this condition has been both fierce and, in certain respects, beside the point; and what the experiences are that millions of people with ADHD find most disabling — experiences that have flooded social media and support communities precisely because official medicine has declined to give them a formal home.

What the Manual Says

DSM-5 defines ADHD as a neurodevelopmental condition characterised by persistent and impairing patterns of inattention and/or hyperactivity-impulsivity. Several additional requirements apply: symptoms must have been present since before the age of twelve; they must occur in at least two settings; they must cause clear functional impairment; and they must not be better explained by another mental disorder.

The inattentive criteria require six or more of the following (five or more for adults over seventeen), present for at least six months at a level inconsistent with developmental stage: failing to give close attention to details or making careless mistakes; difficulty sustaining attention in tasks or play; appearing not to listen when spoken to directly; failing to follow through on instructions and not completing tasks; difficulty organising tasks and activities; avoiding or disliking tasks requiring sustained mental effort; losing things necessary for tasks; being easily distracted by extraneous stimuli; and being forgetful in daily activities.

The hyperactive-impulsive criteria require six or more of the following (again, five for older adolescents and adults): fidgeting or squirming; leaving one's seat when remaining seated is expected; running about or climbing inappropriately (in adults, a subjective sense of restlessness); being unable to play or engage in activities quietly; being 'on the go' as if driven by a motor; talking excessively; blurting out answers before questions are completed; having difficulty waiting one's turn; and interrupting or intruding on others.

Three clinical presentations are recognised. Combined (both inattentive and hyperactive-impulsive criteria met), Predominantly Inattentive (inattention without significant hyperactivity), and Predominantly Hyperactive-Impulsive (the rarer presentation where hyperactivity dominates). Since symptoms shift over time, individuals may move between presentations at different life stages — which is one reason DSM-5 replaced 'subtypes' with 'presentations.'

Laid out like this, the criteria appear systematic and rigorous. Look more closely, and a central challenge emerges immediately.

The Problem the Criteria Cannot Solve

Every symptom on the DSM-5 ADHD list describes something that every human being does, at some frequency, in some circumstances. Everyone loses their keys. Everyone zones out in meetings. Every child fidgets; every teenager interrupts; every adult occasionally forgets what they walked into a room for. The diagnostic task is not to identify these behaviours — it is to determine when they occur with sufficient frequency, severity, and pervasiveness to constitute clinically significant impairment.

This is a judgment call. An important one, and often a well-informed one. But it is not an objective measurement. There is no blood test for ADHD. There is no neuroimaging scan that confirms or refutes the diagnosis. There is no biological marker with the sensitivity and specificity we would expect from a diagnostic test for, say, hypothyroidism or anaemia — both of which, incidentally, can produce attentional symptoms that are clinically indistinguishable from ADHD.

Thomas Insel, former director of the United States National Institute of Mental Health, made this point explicitly in 2013 — a statement remarkable for coming from the head of the institution that funds the majority of psychiatric research: 'While DSM has been described as a Bible for the field, it is, at best, a dictionary. The weakness is its lack of validity. Unlike our definitions of ischemic heart disease, lymphoma, or AIDS, the DSM diagnoses are based on a consensus about clusters of clinical symptoms, not any objective laboratory measure' (Insel, 2013).

Allen Frances, who chaired the DSM-IV task force — the person most directly responsible for the diagnostic criteria that governed ADHD assessment through the 1990s and 2000s — has written that psychiatric diagnoses are 'no more than descriptions of what clinicians observe people do or say, not at all well-established diseases' (Frances, 2013). A 2019 study from the University of Liverpool, published in Psychiatry Research, concluded that diagnostic labels in psychiatry 'create the illusion of an explanation' while providing almost no actionable biological information (Allsopp et al., 2019).

None of this means ADHD is not real. It is. The suffering it causes is real and well-documented. None of it means that clinical diagnosis is pointless — it serves important practical functions. What it means is that the label, on its own, tells you what category the person fits, and very little about the specific neurobiology driving their difficulties. Two people with identical DSM presentations and the same diagnosis may have completely different EEG patterns, different neurochemistry, different nutritional profiles, and different optimal treatment pathways. The diagnosis opens the door. The brain provides the map.

Three Perspectives — Each Containing a Piece of the Truth

The debate about ADHD has taken on the character of a culture war, with positions hardening into camps that talk past each other at considerable volume. In reality, most viewpoints cluster around three broad positions, each of which reflects genuine evidence and genuine limitations. Understanding all three is more clinically useful than endorsing any one of them.

Position One: ADHD is a real, heritable neurodevelopmental disorder — and probably underdiagnosed

The mainstream position in psychiatry and neuroscience holds that ADHD is a well-established neurodevelopmental condition with substantial biological underpinning, and that the dramatic increase in diagnoses reflects improved recognition of a condition that was historically overlooked rather than manufactured concern about normal behaviour.

The evidence base here is solid. Twin and family studies consistently find heritability of 70–80%, making ADHD one of the most heritable of all behavioural traits — more heritable than many purely physical conditions (Faraone & Larsson, 2019). Neuroimaging has identified consistent differences in multiple brain regions: the prefrontal cortex, basal ganglia, anterior cingulate cortex, and cerebellum, all central to attention regulation and executive control. The landmark genome-wide association study (GWAS) by Demontis et al. (2019), the largest genetic analysis of ADHD ever conducted, identified twelve genome-wide significant loci — specific genetic locations where variation reliably predicts ADHD risk. Longitudinal MRI data have found that the prefrontal cortex matures an average of three years later in children with ADHD than in typically developing peers (Shaw et al., 2007). And the functional consequences — academic failure, elevated accident rates, relationship breakdown, substance misuse, reduced life expectancy in severe untreated cases — are documented across decades of follow-up research.

The clinical implication of delayed cortical maturation deserves emphasis. At age seven, when school systems require children to sit still, sustain attention, and self-regulate for extended periods, a seven-year-old with ADHD may have the prefrontal regulatory capacity of a four-year-old. This child is not choosing to misbehave. The circuitry that would allow them to comply is not yet built. Understanding this does not make managing Liam's classroom behaviour any simpler — but it radically changes the moral framing of the problem.

Position Two: ADHD is real but overdiagnosed and overtreated

A second group of clinicians and researchers accepts that ADHD is a genuine condition but believes the diagnostic net has widened considerably beyond what the underlying neurobiology justifies — and that the consequences of this expansion are being inadequately examined.

The most striking empirical evidence here is the relative age effect. Across multiple countries — Germany, Canada, Australia, Taiwan, Denmark, the United States — studies consistently find that the youngest children in a school year cohort are significantly more likely to be diagnosed with ADHD and prescribed stimulant medication than the oldest. In British Columbia, the youngest boys were 30% more likely to receive a diagnosis than the oldest; the youngest girls 70% more likely (Morrow et al., 2012). These children are not disordered. They are younger — less mature developmentally, because of course they are — and that developmental immaturity is being misread as pathology with remarkable consistency across very different healthcare systems.

Kazda et al. (2022), using longitudinal data from a large Australian cohort, found that adolescents diagnosed with ADHD in childhood fared significantly worse on multiple wellbeing measures — including psychological sense of school membership, academic self-concept, and self-efficacy — compared to matched peers with identical behavioural profiles who had not received a diagnosis. This is not simply an argument about overdiagnosis. It is evidence that the diagnostic label itself, under some circumstances, may carry costs that are not acknowledged in the clinical conversation about its benefits.

What makes overdiagnosis particularly difficult to address is that the diagnostic process itself provides almost no safeguard against it. A checklist completed by a teacher who finds a child exhausting, scored against age-norms derived from populations with different demographics, administered in a single clinical encounter without any objective neurophysiological measurement, produces a binary outcome: diagnosis or no diagnosis. It cannot detect the relative age effect. It cannot distinguish developmental immaturity from neurological disorder. It cannot identify the child whose attentional difficulties resolve entirely when a sleep disorder is treated, or the gifted child who is simply understimulated. The tools were not designed to make these distinctions — and in the absence of tools that can, the expanding diagnostic criteria will continue to capture an expanding proportion of the population, not all of whom are genuinely disordered in any meaningful neurobiological sense.

Position Three: ADHD describes behaviours, not a disease — and the description needs revision

The most intellectually ambitious position holds that 'ADHD' as currently defined is a descriptive label applied to a heterogeneous collection of brain states that share surface-level behavioural features but differ substantially in their underlying neurobiology — and that treating them as a single disorder, with a single first-line treatment, is a category error with clinical consequences.

This view is increasingly the dominant one in neurophysiological research. The Demontis et al. (2019) GWAS found that clinical ADHD represents 'an extreme expression of continuous heritable traits' rather than a categorically distinct biological condition. Richard Saul, a behavioural neurologist with decades of clinical experience, documented over twenty conditions — including thyroid disorders, iron deficiency anaemia, sleep disorders, anxiety, giftedness, and vision impairments — whose primary presentation could meet DSM criteria for ADHD. His conclusion — that 'ADHD does not exist' — overstates the case for rhetorical impact. His underlying observation — that the same symptom cluster arises from multiple distinct biological mechanisms, and that the DSM label does nothing to distinguish between them — is empirically defensible and clinically important (Saul, 2014).

Our own view, shaped by years of clinical work and by the neurophysiological data accessible through QEEG, is that all three positions contain something true — and that the argument has persisted so long partly because each camp is examining a different part of the same problem. ADHD is real. It is heterogeneous. Its symptoms exist on a continuum. The same behavioural presentation can arise from multiple biological mechanisms. And those mechanisms matter enormously — because they determine what will actually help.

The Bell Curve and the Neurodiversity Question

Most psychological traits are normally distributed across the population. Attention span, like blood pressure, like height, like processing speed, follows a bell curve — most people cluster around the mean, smaller numbers fall toward the extremes. There is no clear biological break between 'normal' attention and 'disordered' attention. The diagnostic threshold is a line drawn on a continuum, in a location chosen by committee, revised periodically by subsequent committees.

The neurodiversity framework — the idea that variations in brain function, including those associated with ADHD, represent natural human variation rather than pathological defect — has gained significant cultural traction, and not without reason. It shifts the question from 'what is wrong with this person?' to 'what environment would allow this brain to function at its best?' — a reframing with genuine clinical utility.

But neurodiversity as a complete clinical framework has limits. It works well for Oliver, whose rigidity and hyperfocus become assets in the right context, and for entrepreneurs whose novelty-seeking and risk tolerance translate into genuine professional advantage. It works less well for Daniel, who cannot finish anything regardless of context, or for Maya, whose emotional responses cause her suffering that is independent of her environment, or for Liam, whose trajectory without appropriate understanding and intervention is heading toward places he has not chosen. The neurodiversity lens and the medical treatment lens are not incompatible — but conflating them can obscure the very real need for intervention when that need is present.

The Symptoms Nobody Put in the Manual

Walk into any ADHD support group, online community, or TikTok comment section and you will encounter a vocabulary that does not appear anywhere in the DSM-5. These terms have proliferated because they describe experiences that millions of people with ADHD report as central to their daily difficulty — experiences that official psychiatry, in its focus on observable and categorizable behaviours, has not formalised. We want to be transparent about these symptoms: the evidence base varies, some constructs are better supported than others, and not all of them are specific to ADHD. But dismissing them because they have not been through a DSM committee would be both intellectually lazy and clinically unkind.

Rejection Sensitive Dysphoria

The term Rejection Sensitive Dysphoria (RSD), coined and popularised by the American ADHD specialist William Dodson, describes an intense, near-physical emotional pain triggered by perceived rejection, criticism, failure, or teasing — even when the trigger is minor, ambiguous, or entirely imagined. People with RSD describe a sudden, overwhelming emotional flood that feels completely disproportionate to the situation: a critical comment from a colleague, an unreturned text message, a tone of voice that reads as cool. For many adults with ADHD — particularly those with limbic and inattentive presentations — RSD is experienced as one of their most disabling features.

The scientific caveat: RSD as a discrete construct has not been formally validated in peer-reviewed research to the standard of the core DSM criteria. There is no agreed diagnostic threshold. The proposed neurological basis — involving heightened amygdalar reactivity and possibly noradrenergic dysregulation — is plausible and consistent with what we know about emotional regulation in ADHD but remains insufficiently studied. Many researchers prefer to frame the phenomenon as a manifestation of the emotional dysregulation that is well-documented in ADHD, rather than a separate construct with its own name.

Our clinical view: the phenomenon is real, and it is sufficiently common and sufficiently impairing to deserve clinical attention regardless of what we call it. Many people with ADHD have spent decades being told they are 'too sensitive,' 'overreacting,' or 'making a big deal out of nothing.' Understanding this as a neurological feature rather than a personality failing does not make it less painful — but it changes the therapeutic approach, and it changes the conversation.

Time Blindness

Russell Barkley, one of the world's most influential ADHD researchers, has argued that the central deficit in ADHD is not attention per se but self-regulation across time. His concept of 'time blindness' describes an impaired internal sense of time passing: difficulty estimating how long tasks will take, an inability to feel the approach of future events with the urgency that those events objectively deserve, and a lived experience dominated by two temporal zones — 'now' and 'not now' (Barkley, 2012).

In practice, this manifests as the pattern that puzzles everyone who knows someone with ADHD: things exist, neurologically, only when they are immediately present or about to produce a crisis. The deadline three weeks away does not register with the same weight as the deadline three hours away. The tax return, the promised phone call, the appointment that needs rescheduling — these dissolve into unreality the moment they pass out of immediate view, to reappear with sudden and vivid urgency when the crisis is imminent.

This is not procrastination in the colloquial sense of choosing to avoid an unpleasant task. It is a genuine difference in how time is internally represented and experienced — one that has neurobiological correlates in the dopamine-dependent reward prediction systems of the prefrontal cortex. Understanding it this way changes the interventions: external structure, deadlines imposed from outside the self, body-doubling, and calendar-based accountability systems are not crutches for the weak-willed. They are prosthetic time-awareness for a brain whose internal time-keeping machinery is calibrated differently.

Hyperfocus — The Superpower With a Sharp Edge

The name 'Attention Deficit' is, in the context of hyperfocus, spectacularly misleading. ADHD does not produce an absence of attention. It produces dysregulated attention — which means it can swing in either direction. Hyperfocus is the capacity to become so completely absorbed in an engaging task that time, hunger, social obligations, and other people's needs cease to register. It is the mechanism by which Oliver can spend six unbroken hours on a structural engineering problem that genuinely interests him, and then find it literally impossible to spend twenty minutes on a performance review that doesn't.

Neurologically, this is a story about dopamine and salience. The ADHD brain's reward-prediction machinery tends to assign insufficient salience to important-but-uninteresting tasks and excessive salience to novel, immediately stimulating ones. When a task provides sufficient dopaminergic activation — through novelty, urgency, genuine interest, or competitive pressure — the ADHD brain can produce sustained focus that surpasses that of neurotypical peers. When it doesn't, no amount of effort can reliably manufacture that focus from scratch.

Hyperfocus looks like a superpower when directed at the right target. It looks like a disaster — missed meals, failed relationships, ignored responsibilities — when it isn't. The person with ADHD is not choosing which target it lands on. Their brain is running a reward calculation over which they have limited conscious control, and arriving at answers that don't always serve them.

Emotional Dysregulation — The Most Consequential Omission

Perhaps the single most clinically significant thing missing from the DSM-5 ADHD criteria is emotional dysregulation — the difficulty many people with ADHD experience in managing the speed, intensity, and duration of their emotional responses. This is not simply being irritable or short-tempered. It is a neurological pattern in which emotions arrive faster, feel more intense, and take longer to dissipate than they do in neurotypical individuals — and in which the gap between feeling an emotion and expressing it is narrower than most social and professional environments can accommodate without consequence.

Barkley and colleagues have estimated that emotional dysregulation is present in up to 70% of adults with ADHD and may account for more functional impairment in adult populations than the core attentional symptoms — more failed relationships, more lost jobs, more sustained suffering — than inattention or hyperactivity alone (Barkley, 2010). It is the feature most consistently associated with poor quality of life in adult ADHD, and the feature most consistently absent from standard treatment plans.

Its exclusion from the DSM criteria was partly a consequence of its overlap with mood disorders — the diagnostic committee's concern about false positives — and partly a reflection of the DSM's tendency to privilege reliability (consistent identification between clinicians) over comprehensiveness (accurate capture of the full clinical picture). The result is that emotional dysregulation in ADHD is undertreated, underrecognised, and disproportionately responsible for the outcomes that make ADHD genuinely debilitating in adult life. Maya's entire clinical history — sixteen years of treatment for downstream emotional consequences while the upstream driver went unaddressed — is a case study in this omission.

What the Diagnosis Gives You — and What It Doesn't

An ADHD diagnosis, at its best, opens access to educational accommodations, workplace adjustments, and appropriate treatment. It provides a framework — however imperfect — for understanding a pattern of difficulties. It connects people to communities of shared experience and validated recognition, which for many individuals is the first time in their lives that someone has not simply told them to try harder.

What it does not provide is an explanation. It does not tell you which neural system is primarily implicated, why that system is dysregulated in this particular person, or what specifically will help. The same diagnosis encompasses Oliver's rigid hyperfocus, Liam's impulsive hyperactivity, Zara's sensory overload, and Priya's quiet drift — four completely different neurological patterns, all labelled with the same four letters, all potentially receiving the same first-line treatment.

This is the central problem this book exists to address. Not to argue about whether ADHD is real — it is — but to insist that the real question is not 'does this person have ADHD?' but 'what is happening in this person's brain, and what does that tell us about what will actually help them?'

To answer that question, we need to go deeper than the symptom list. In the next chapter, we explore the full clinical territory that surrounds the ADHD diagnosis: the conditions that travel with it, the conditions that masquerade as it, the ways in which our current approach systematically fails certain populations, and why the diagnostic trap of symptom overlap is considerably more consequential than is generally acknowledged.

References — Chapter Two

Insel, T. (2013). 'Transforming diagnosis.' Director's Blog, National Institute of Mental Health.

Frances, A. (2013). 'The past, present and future of psychiatric diagnosis.' World Psychiatry, 12(2), 99–105.

Allsopp, K., Read, J., Corcoran, R. & Kinderman, P. (2019). 'Heterogeneity in psychiatric diagnostic classification.' Psychiatry Research, 279, 15–22.

Faraone, S.V. & Larsson, H. (2019). 'Genetics of attention deficit hyperactivity disorder.' Molecular Psychiatry, 24(4), 562–575.

Demontis, D. et al. (2019). 'Discovery of the first genome-wide significant risk loci for ADHD.' Nature Genetics, 51(1), 63–75.

Shaw, P. et al. (2007). 'ADHD is characterized by a delay in cortical maturation.' PNAS, 104(49), 19649–19654.

Morrow, R.L. et al. (2012). 'Influence of relative age on diagnosis and treatment of ADHD.' CMAJ, 184(7), 755–762.

Kazda, L. et al. (2022). 'Association of ADHD diagnosis with adolescent quality of life.' JAMA Network Open, 5(10), e2236364.

Saul, R. (2014). ADHD Does Not Exist. New York: HarperCollins.

Barkley, R.A. (2010). 'Deficient emotional self-regulation: a core component of ADHD.' Journal of ADHD & Related Disorders, 1(2), 5–37.

Barkley, R.A. (2012). Executive Functions: What They Are, How They Work, and Why They Evolved. New York: Guilford Press.

Dodson, W. (2016). 'Emotional regulation and rejection sensitive dysphoria.' ADDitude Magazine.

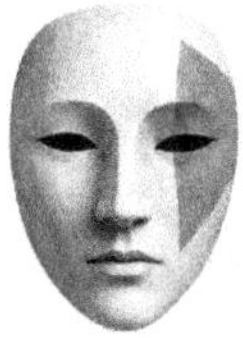

Chapter Three
The Overlapping Universe

ADHD, comorbidities, mimics, and the art of missing the point

> ***MAYA — Age 32:*** *She has seen a psychiatrist for depression (three antidepressants), a therapist for anxiety (two CBT courses), a GP for chronic insomnia (a sleep hygiene leaflet and a referral to a waiting list), a gastroenterologist for IBS that nobody has connected to anything else, and briefly — at her mother's increasingly desperate suggestion — a nutritionist. She is 32, she is exhausted, and she is still unable to finish a task without it becoming a crisis or start one without it becoming an ordeal. Nobody has connected the dots. Nobody has looked at her brain.*

If ADHD were a clean, bounded diagnosis — a single condition with defined edges, a specific biological cause, and a corresponding treatment — the clinical picture would be straightforward. Identify the symptoms. Make the diagnosis. Prescribe the treatment. Monitor. Adjust. Discharge when stable.

It is not. And the consequences of pretending otherwise have been playing out, largely unacknowledged, in clinics around the world for decades.

ADHD is one of the most comorbid conditions in all of psychiatry. Between 60% and 80% of individuals with the diagnosis have at least one additional diagnosable condition — many have two or three (Jensen & Steinhausen, 2015; Brown, 2009). The comorbidities range from anxiety disorders and mood disorders to sleep disorders, learning disabilities, autism spectrum conditions, substance use disorders, and personality disorders. Their relationship to ADHD is rarely simple: sometimes the ADHD drives the comorbidity (years of attentional failure producing a chronic low-grade despair that meets criteria for major depression), sometimes the comorbidity produces the attentional symptoms (a brain in a state of chronic threat-detection has very limited capacity for sustained cognitive focus), and sometimes both arise from shared underlying neurobiological architecture.

Disentangling these possibilities requires more than a symptom checklist and a clinical interview. It requires looking at the brain.

The Conditions That Travel With ADHD

Anxiety: When the Same Symptoms Mean Opposite Things

Anxiety disorders co-occur with ADHD in approximately 50% of affected individuals (Brown, 2009). This co-occurrence rate should give any prescribing clinician pause, because the distinction between anxiety-driven and ADHD-driven attentional difficulties has profound implications for treatment — and because that distinction cannot be made from a symptom checklist.

Consider what a brain in a state of anxious overarousal looks like: distractible, unable to sustain focus on the task at hand, prone to jumping between thoughts, emotionally reactive, physically restless. Now consider what a brain in a state of cortical underactivation looks like: distractible, unable to sustain focus, prone to mind-wandering, emotionally variable, physically restless. On a behavioural rating scale, these two profiles are nearly identical. In terms of what is actually happening neurologically, they are polar opposites.

The overaroused anxious brain is running too fast — too much high-frequency activity, too much threat-detection, too much internal noise. The underactivated ADHD brain is running too slowly — insufficient frontal activation, a reward-prediction system that cannot generate enough motivational drive for sustained effort. Stimulant medications, which are first-line for ADHD, increase cortical arousal. Applied to the underactivated brain, this helps. Applied to the already overaroused anxious brain, it commonly produces worsening anxiety, disrupted sleep, increased irritability, and occasionally panic — outcomes that, in the absence of any neurophysiological measurement, are difficult to predict and are too often attributed to medication dosing rather than to an incorrect treatment selection.

Quantitative EEG distinguishes these profiles. A clinical interview, however thorough, cannot do so reliably. This is not a limitation of the clinician's skill. It is a limitation of the tool.

Depression: The Accumulated Weight of a Mismatched Brain

Major depression co-occurs with ADHD in approximately 38% of adults with the diagnosis (Kessler et al., 2006). In many cases — perhaps most — the depression is not a separate, independent disease that happens to accompany the ADHD. It is the emotional residue of a lifetime of underperforming in systems designed for a different kind of brain.

Repeat this experience enough times — trying hard and still failing, being told you're not working hard enough when you are in fact working twice as hard for half the result, watching relationships deteriorate partly because of things you couldn't control, missing opportunities because the time-blindness swallowed them — and the emotional consequence is a characteristic despair that looks like major depression because, functionally and phenomenologically, it is. It responds, partially, to antidepressants. It does not resolve without addressing the ADHD that is producing it.

Maya's clinical history is the textbook version of this failure mode: sixteen years of treatment for downstream emotional consequences, while the upstream neurological driver was never assessed, never measured, and never directly addressed. Each of her treating clinicians was competent. Each made reasonable decisions based on the information available to them. None of them had access to the information that would have changed the approach — because accessing that information requires looking at the brain, which none of them did.

Sleep Disorders: The Most Underestimated Engine

Sleep problems are present in 73–78% of children with ADHD and appear to be even more prevalent in adults (Cortese et al., 2013). The relationship is bidirectional, clinically important, and systematically underappreciated.

Chronic sleep deprivation produces a symptom cluster that is clinically indistinguishable from ADHD: impaired sustained attention, degraded working memory, emotional lability, increased impulsivity, and slowed processing speed. A child whose classroom behaviour is driven primarily by sleep-disordered breathing — obstruction during sleep producing intermittent hypoxia and fragmented sleep architecture — will score in the diagnostic range on every standardised ADHD rating scale while having no ADHD-specific pathology. The treatment for their attentional difficulties is an ENT referral, not a stimulant prescription. These cases are common. They are routinely mismanaged.

Richard Saul documented sleep disorders as among the most frequent conditions he found underlying apparent ADHD in his clinical practice — a finding consistent with what any clinician who takes a systematic sleep history will discover (Saul, 2014). Sleep disorders and ADHD also co-occur frequently: restless legs syndrome, delayed sleep phase disorder, and sleep apnoea are all more prevalent in ADHD populations than in the general population, creating presentations where both conditions are present and both need addressing. The standard ADHD assessment process does not include a systematic sleep evaluation. It should.

Autism Spectrum Disorder: The Boundary That Should Not Have Existed

Until DSM-5 was published in 2013, clinicians were explicitly instructed not to diagnose ADHD in individuals with autism spectrum disorder. This prohibition was a clinical fiction that persisted for decades: the two conditions co-occur in approximately 30–50% of cases (Leitner, 2014), they share genetic architecture (Demontis et al., 2019 confirmed significant genetic correlations between ADHD and ASD risk variants), and they share neurophysiological patterns that create genuine diagnostic complexity — particularly in girls and women, where both conditions characteristically present more subtly and are consequently more systematically missed.

DSM-5 corrected the prohibition in principle. Clinical practice has been slower to update, and many practitioners still default to a single primary diagnosis rather than recognising and treating overlapping presentations simultaneously. The co-occurrence of ADHD and ASD — increasingly recognised under the term

AuDHD — is more prevalent than clinical practice typically reflects. A 2021 meta-analysis of over fifty studies found that 39% of people with ASD also met criteria for ADHD; a 2024 school-population study found that 33% of children with ADHD also had ASD, yet only 16% of those with both conditions had received both diagnoses (Canals et al., 2024; Ying et al., 2021). This matters because the co-occurring conditions interact: anxiety secondary to ASD-related social difficulty looks different from anxiety secondary to ADHD-related emotional dysregulation, and requires different interventions. Treating them as the same thing — because the rating scale doesn't distinguish between them — is a clinical shortcut with predictable consequences.

Substance Use: Self-Medication and Shared Biology

Adults with ADHD have substantially and consistently elevated rates of alcohol and drug use disorders. The mechanisms are multiple. Some substance use represents deliberate, often partially effective, self-medication of intolerable symptoms — cannabis for the anxiety and internal noise, stimulants for the cognitive difficulties, alcohol for the emotional dysregulation and sleep difficulties. Some represents the consequence of impulsivity and reduced executive inhibition lowering the barrier to substance initiation in adolescence. And some reflects shared genetic vulnerability: the Demontis GWAS study (2019) found positive genetic correlations between ADHD risk and tobacco use, alcohol dependence, and substance use disorders — indicating these are not independent conditions that happen to co-occur but conditions that share some of their biological foundations.

The Satterfield et al. (2007) thirty-year follow-up of hyperactive boys found that even intensive multimodality treatment in childhood — medication plus years of psychological and educational intervention — did not prevent elevated rates of adult criminality and substance misuse. The risk was not eliminated by treating the ADHD. This is one of the most consequential and least cited findings in the ADHD literature: it points to an underlying biological vulnerability that symptomatic treatment of the attention and impulse symptoms does not adequately address. Understanding and targeting that underlying vulnerability — through the brain-based approach this book advocates — is not supplementary care. It is the point.

ADHD and Complex PTSD — The Diagnostic Confusion Nobody Warns You About

Of all the conditions that overlap with ADHD, Complex Post-Traumatic Stress Disorder (C-PTSD) represents one of the most clinically consequential and least formally studied diagnostic challenges. C-PTSD — recognised in the ICD-11 as a distinct condition arising from prolonged or repeated trauma, and characterised by the core PTSD symptoms plus three additional disturbances of self-organisation: emotional dysregulation, negative self-concept, and interpersonal difficulties — shares a striking number of surface features with ADHD. Inattention, difficulty concentrating, emotional dysregulation, impulsivity, hyperarousal, sleep disruption, and impaired executive function appear in both. The hyperarousal of C-PTSD is behaviourally indistinguishable from the hyperactivity of ADHD on standard rating scales. The profound difficulties with emotional regulation that characterise C-PTSD — the rapid, overwhelming shifts in affect, the chronic negative self-perception, the relational instability — overlap substantially with the emotional dysregulation, rejection sensitivity, and interpersonal difficulty documented in ADHD. The assessment checklist sees the same surface regardless of which condition is driving it.

It is important to acknowledge that the specific research literature on C-PTSD and ADHD overlap remains limited, largely because C-PTSD only received formal ICD-11 recognition in 2022 and the DSM-5 does not include it as a discrete diagnosis. The broader PTSD and ADHD literature, however, provides a relevant foundation. A 2023 systematic review in the Journal of Neuroscience Research confirmed that attentional dysfunction in PTSD is common and clinically significant, and that impaired sustained attention is not specific to ADHD (Fleurkens et al., 2023). Studies using PTSD criteria have found co-occurrence rates with ADHD of approximately 10% — compared to 1.6% in the general population — and that ADHD itself is an independent risk factor for developing PTSD, with impulsivity, poor boundary recognition, and chronic adversity all increasing trauma vulnerability (Adler et al., 2004). When both conditions are present, each amplifies the other: trauma worsens attentional and executive function difficulties, while ADHD-related impulsivity and emotional intensity complicate trauma recovery. As C-PTSD-specific research develops, clinical experience strongly suggests that the diagnostic confusion will prove to be at least as significant as — and possibly greater than — the already documented PTSD/ADHD overlap, given that C-PTSD's disturbances of self-organisation map so directly onto ADHD's most impairing and most frequently misattributed features. For any individual presenting with a complex trauma history alongside attentional and regulatory difficulties, assessment for both conditions — rather than assignment to a single diagnostic box — is clinically essential.

When What Looks Like ADHD Isn't

Richard Saul's clinical provocation — that 'ADHD does not exist' — overstates the case, as it was designed to. His underlying observation is important: the DSM-5 diagnostic criteria are sufficiently non-specific that they can be met by individuals with a wide range of conditions that are not ADHD and that respond to treatments that are entirely different from those used for ADHD.

In fifty years of clinical practice in behavioural neurology, Saul identified more than twenty such conditions. They include thyroid disorders — both hyper- and hypothyroidism produce attentional impairment that resolves with thyroid normalisation; iron deficiency anaemia — the relationship between low ferritin and attentional function is well-established, and iron supplementation in iron-deficient children produces measurable improvements in sustained attention and working memory; vision and hearing impairments — a child who cannot see the board clearly or cannot hear the teacher reliably will have attentional difficulties that are sensory rather than neurological in origin; sleep disorders; generalised anxiety; depression; obsessive-compulsive disorder; giftedness in unstimulating educational environments; and several less common conditions including lead toxicity, coeliac disease, and certain metabolic disorders (Saul, 2014).

The clinical implication is not that ADHD is fictional. It is that a diagnostic process that relies solely on symptom observation — without any objective assessment of the biological systems that might be driving those symptoms — will systematically misdiagnose a proportion of patients, prescribe treatments that are at best ineffective and at worst harmful, and miss conditions that are often more straightforward to treat than ADHD itself. Treating iron deficiency anaemia is safer than prescribing amphetamines. Treating sleep-disordered breathing is more effective than managing the attentional symptoms it produces. These are not alternative medicine. They are basic medical workup that the current diagnostic pathway does not require.

The Diagnostic Trap of Symptom Overlap

Five symptoms: difficulty concentrating, restlessness, irritability, sleep disturbance, and impulsivity. This cluster appears in ADHD. It also appears in generalised anxiety disorder, major depressive disorder, bipolar disorder, post-traumatic stress disorder, thyroid disorders, iron deficiency, chronic sleep deprivation, and in any person who is working in an environment profoundly mismatched to their cognitive style, under conditions of significant chronic stress.

The University of Liverpool's 2019 analysis, published in Psychiatry Research, found 'a huge amount of overlap in symptoms between diagnoses' across the DSM's five major diagnostic chapters and concluded that the categorical system 'creates the illusion of an explanation' while providing almost no actionable biological information (Allsopp et al., 2019). This is not a criticism of individual clinicians. It is a structural problem with a diagnostic system built to maximise consistency between clinicians rather than correspondence between labels and biological reality.

The practical consequence: a person presenting with attentional difficulties to a psychiatrist who specialises in anxiety is more likely to receive an anxiety diagnosis. The same person presenting to one who specialises in mood disorders is more likely to receive a depression diagnosis. The same person presenting to an ADHD specialist is more likely to receive an ADHD diagnosis. None of these clinicians is necessarily wrong — the comorbidities are real and all may be present. But none of them can answer, from a symptom checklist, the question that actually determines optimal treatment: what is the specific neurophysiological pattern driving these symptoms in this specific brain, and what does that tell us about what will actually help?

The Gender Blindspot — How a Diagnosis Was Built Around the Wrong Child

The history of ADHD research is, in substantial part, a history of studying boys and generalising the findings to everyone.

The early clinical descriptions — Still, Kramer and Pollnow, Bradley — were dominated by boys. The research populations used to develop and validate diagnostic criteria were majority male. The hyperactive, impulsive, disruptive boy became the clinical prototype against which all ADHD presentations were measured. The quiet, inattentive, internally struggling girl became invisible, because she didn't match the template — and because her inattention was silent, her distress private, and her compliance sufficiently adequate that no one in the school or clinic felt the urgency to investigate further.

Women and girls with ADHD are consistently more likely than their male counterparts to: present with inattentive rather than combined presentations; develop sophisticated compensatory strategies that mask their deficits publicly while exacting a substantial private cognitive and emotional toll; present to clinical settings with anxiety or depression as the primary complaint; and be diagnosed with a mood disorder before — or instead of — an attention disorder (Quinn & Madhoo, 2014). The research is increasingly documenting the role of oestrogen in modulating dopaminergic function, with ADHD symptoms worsening significantly around menstruation, perimenopause, and menopause in women who may have appeared relatively well-compensated during their reproductive years.

Priya will wait years longer for an accurate assessment than Liam. Not because she is less affected by her attentional differences — she is arguably more affected in certain domains — but because the system was built to find Liam and not her. A diagnostic process whose primary tools are rating scales completed by teachers who are relieved to have a quiet student is not a diagnostic process that will find the quiet student's problem. This is a design flaw in the assessment system, not an inherent property of the condition, and it is correctable — but only if we are willing to add objective measures that do not depend on how disruptive the patient is.

Why Comorbidity Changes Everything

The clinical implications of ADHD's comorbidity profile are frequently underestimated in ways that have direct consequences for patients. They mean the most effective treatment is almost never a single intervention targeting only ADHD symptoms. They mean that what looks like treatment failure may be an untreated co-occurring condition generating residual symptoms. They mean the order in which conditions are prioritised matters: treating severe sleep disorder first may resolve what appeared to be ADHD; treating ADHD without addressing chronic anxiety may produce a patient who is marginally less distracted and considerably more agitated.

They also mean — most consequentially — that operating without objective neurophysiological data in a condition with known and substantial heterogeneity is making treatment decisions with a fundamentally incomplete picture. The symptoms are visible. The brain producing them is not. Until we can measure the brain — its specific electrical patterns, its arousal state, its network dynamics, its neurotransmitter balance — we are making inferences from the shadow cast by the object rather than examining the object itself.

In the next chapter, we turn from the shadow to the object. We examine what neuroscience has revealed about the genes, neurotransmitters, and brain networks that underlie attention regulation and its failure — and begin to see why the same diagnostic label genuinely covers different neurological territory in different people.

References — Chapter Three

Brown, T.E. (2009). ADHD Comorbidities: Handbook for ADHD Complications in Children and Adults. Washington DC: American Psychiatric Press.

Jensen, C.M. & Steinhausen, H.C. (2015). 'Comorbid mental disorders in children and adolescents with ADHD in a large nationwide study.' ADHD Attention Deficit and Hyperactivity Disorders, 7, 27–38.

Kessler, R.C. et al. (2006). 'The prevalence and correlates of adult ADHD in the United States.' American Journal of Psychiatry, 163(4), 716–723.

Cortese, S. et al. (2013). 'Sleep in children with attention-deficit/hyperactivity disorder: a meta-analysis.' Sleep Medicine Reviews, 17(4), 287–296.

Leitner, Y. (2014). 'The co-occurrence of autism and ADHD in children.' Frontiers in Human Neuroscience, 8, 268.

Demontis, D. et al. (2019). 'Discovery of the first genome-wide significant risk loci for ADHD.' Nature Genetics, 51(1), 63–75.

Ying, R. et al. (2021). 'Prevalence of attention-deficit/hyperactivity disorder in individuals with autism spectrum disorder: a meta-analysis.' *Research in Autism Spectrum Disorders*, 83, 101759.

Canals, J. et al. (2024). 'Prevalence of comorbidity of autism and ADHD and associated characteristics in school population: EPINED study.' *Autism Research*, 17(5), 1002–1015.

Satterfield, J.H. et al. (2007). 'A 30-year prospective follow-up study of hyperactive boys with conduct problems: adult criminality.' Journal of the American Academy of Child & Adolescent Psychiatry, 46(5), 601–610.

Fleurkens, P. et al. (2023). 'Attention deficits as a key player in the symptomatology of posttraumatic stress disorder: a review.' *Journal of Neuroscience Research*, 101, 1068–1085.

Adler, L.A. et al. (2004). 'Attention-deficit/hyperactivity disorder in adult patients with posttraumatic stress disorder: is ADHD a vulnerability factor?' *Journal of Attention Disorders*, 8(1), 11–16.

Szymanski, K., Sapanski, L. & Conway, F. (2011). 'Trauma and ADHD — association or diagnostic confusion? A clinical perspective.' *Journal of Infant, Child and Adolescent Psychotherapy*, 10(1), 51–59.

World Health Organization. (2022). *International Classification of Diseases, 11th Revision (ICD-11).* Geneva: WHO. [C-PTSD diagnostic criteria: 6B41]

Saul, R. (2014). ADHD Does Not Exist. New York: HarperCollins.

Allsopp, K. et al. (2019). 'Heterogeneity in psychiatric diagnostic classification.' Psychiatry Research, 279, 15–22.

Quinn, P.O. & Madhoo, M. (2014). 'A review of attention-deficit/hyperactivity disorder in women and girls.' Primary Care Companion for CNS Disorders, 16(3).

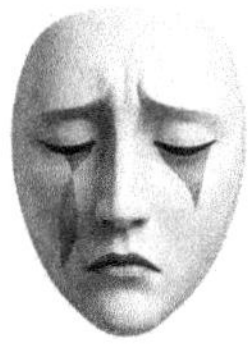

Chapter Four

The Neuroscience of a Wandering Mind

Genes, neurotransmitters, and the brain networks behind ADHD

> ***ZARA — Age 16:*** *Her mother takes her to a neurologist. The MRI is clean. 'There is nothing structurally wrong with your daughter's brain,' the neurologist says, with the satisfaction of someone who has ruled out a tumour and considers the appointment a success. Her mother thanks him. Zara stares at the EEG machine in the corner of the room — unpowered, dusty, unused — and says nothing. There is nothing structurally wrong. Nobody has asked what is functionally wrong. Nobody has asked how the brain is working — only what it looks like sitting still in a scanner.*

Here is the version of ADHD neuroscience that appears in pharmaceutical information leaflets, patient-facing websites, and more clinical consultations than most psychiatrists would feel comfortable acknowledging: the brain isn't making enough dopamine; the medication tops it up; the problem is solved. Neat, mechanistic, satisfying. The chemical imbalance story has proven extraordinarily resilient — not because it is scientifically rigorous, but because it is narratively perfect. It offers a biological explanation that reduces stigma, justifies a pharmacological solution, and can be communicated in under thirty seconds. So thoroughly has it permeated popular culture that dopamine has become the neurochemical of the moment: people speak casually of dopamine hits, dopamine seeking, and dopamine fasting with a confidence that implies they are describing something measurable happening in real time in their own brains. It is worth pausing on the irony here. Dopamine has become perhaps the most discussed neurotransmitter in contemporary culture — and yet no standard ADHD assessment anywhere in the world measures brain dopamine. Not directly. Not indirectly through urinary metabolites. Not through cerebrospinal fluid. The diagnosis that has been built, in the public imagination and in much clinical practice, on the architecture of dopamine deficiency does not include a single objective measure of dopamine as part of its standard workup. This is not merely an academic observation. It is the central epistemological problem with the chemical imbalance framing: a theory sufficiently vague that it cannot be tested, sufficiently compelling that it is rarely questioned, and sufficiently useful — commercially and clinically — that the incentive to question it has never been overwhelming.

It is also incomplete in ways that matter enormously for clinical practice.

The actual neuroscience of ADHD is considerably more complex, considerably more interesting, and considerably more useful — if you are willing to sit with the complexity rather than paper over it. Attention is not a single function controlled by a single neurotransmitter in a single brain region. It is an emergent property of multiple large-scale neural networks, modulated by at least three major neurotransmitter systems, shaped by genetic architecture and epigenetic environment, and profoundly variable between individuals. Understanding why it fails in ADHD — and understanding why it fails differently in different people — requires a brief but genuine tour of the brain's most relevant architecture.

This chapter provides that tour. Not as academic decoration, but as the necessary foundation for everything in Part Two.

Genetics: Strongly Inherited, Complexly Determined

ADHD is among the most heritable of all behavioural conditions. Twin studies consistently find heritability estimates of 70–80%, meaning that roughly three-quarters of the variation in ADHD traits across the population is explained by genetic differences rather than environmental ones (Faraone & Larsson, 2019). In practical terms: when a child receives an ADHD diagnosis, there is a very high probability that a biological parent, sibling, or close relative has either a diagnosis or prominent subclinical traits. ADHD family trees have a characteristic density that experienced clinicians learn to recognise in the first few minutes of a family history.

But heritability is widely misunderstood. It does not mean genetically fixed, developmentally predetermined, or impervious to intervention. It means that genetic factors account for a large proportion of the variation in ADHD traits between individuals in a given population, under observed environmental conditions. The same genetic profile can produce quite different outcomes in different environments — a point of profound practical importance. The ADHD brain is not a broken brain. In significant respects, it is a brain calibrated for an environment different from the one most contemporary schools and offices provide.

The genetic architecture of ADHD is highly polygenic. The landmark Demontis et al. (2019) GWAS meta-analysis — involving over 55,000 individuals, the largest such study of ADHD to date — identified twelve genome-wide significant loci. These include variants near FOXP2 (involved in synapse formation and speech development, and previously associated with language disorders), SORCS3 (a brain-expressed transmembrane receptor important for neuronal plasticity, previously associated with depression and Alzheimer's risk), and DUSP6 (a phosphatase implicated in dopamine transporter function and synaptic regulation). Together, these twelve loci explain only a fraction of the total heritable variance. Thousands of additional common variants, each contributing effects too small to be detected individually, account for the remainder — a pattern that places ADHD firmly in the category of complex polygenic traits, alongside height, intelligence, and cardiovascular disease risk.

The genetic correlation data from the same study deserves particular clinical attention. ADHD shares significant genetic architecture with major depressive disorder (genetic correlation 0.42), educational underattainment (-0.53), obesity-related traits, insomnia, and smoking initiation. These correlations are not confounders. They are indications that the genetic factors underlying ADHD influence biological systems extending well beyond attentional regulation — including reward processing, metabolic function, and sleep architecture — all of which are directly relevant to comprehensive assessment and treatment.

Pineda-Cirera et al. (2019), using a novel approach to identify genetic variants that influence DNA methylation specifically in human brain tissue, added an epigenetic dimension to this picture. They found that ADHD risk variants are enriched in regions of allele-specific methylation — meaning genetic risk for ADHD influences which genes are switched on and off in specific brain regions. The genes identified include ARTN, which supports the survival of dopaminergic neurons in the ventral midbrain, and PIDD1, a cell life regulator. These findings illustrate that ADHD, at the molecular level, involves biological complexity that a symptom checklist cannot begin to capture — and that nutritional and environmental factors capable of influencing DNA methylation may represent genuine treatment targets.

Neurotransmitters: A More Complicated Story Than the Leaflets Suggest

Dopamine — Not a Deficit, But a Dysregulation

Dopamine's role in ADHD is genuine, well-documented, and clinically important. But the 'dopamine deficit model' — the idea that ADHD brains produce insufficient dopamine and stimulants correct this deficiency in the way that insulin corrects a deficit in diabetes — is substantially oversimplified.

Dopamine's primary function is not producing pleasure. It is predicting reward, calibrating the motivational weight of effort, and regulating the drive to initiate and sustain goal-directed behaviour. Disrupted dopaminergic signalling in the mesocortical pathway — from the ventral tegmental area to the prefrontal cortex — reduces the brain's ability to assign adequate motivational weight to effortful tasks that lack immediate payoff. The consequence is not a general cognitive failure but a motivational calibration problem: the brain runs a reward calculation and consistently arrives at answers that don't favour tasks that are important but not immediately stimulating.

The del Campo et al. (2013) PET study, using 18F-fallypride imaging in adults with ADHD and matched controls, produced a finding that complicated the standard narrative considerably.

There were no significant group differences in D2/D3 dopamine receptor availability between ADHD patients and controls as a whole. Instead, poor attentional performers — drawn from both groups — showed significantly reduced dopamine activity in the left caudate nucleus. Methylphenidate improved attention in a baseline-performance-dependent manner regardless of diagnosis: it helped low performers and was ineffective or mildly detrimental for high performers, irrespective of whether they had ADHD. The authors concluded that 'dopamine dysregulation per se is unlikely to be the primary cause underlying ADHD pathology in adults' — a conclusion with significant implications for how we conceptualise and communicate the mechanism of stimulant treatment to patients.

Stimulants increase synaptic dopamine availability — that part of the mechanism is accurate. But they do not specifically target a brain that has too little dopamine. They increase dopamine availability in a way that improves performance in some cognitive profiles and not others, and that has nothing specifically to do with whether the person meets diagnostic criteria for ADHD. The symptom checklist cannot predict who will benefit. The brain's neurophysiological profile can.

Noradrenaline — The Signal Sharpener and the Stress Amplifier

Noradrenaline, produced primarily in the locus coeruleus — a small, intensely concentrated cluster of neurons in the brainstem that projects widely across the cortex — regulates arousal and performs signal-to-noise optimisation in prefrontal networks. When noradrenergic tone is optimal, the prefrontal cortex is well-tuned: relevant stimuli are amplified, irrelevant stimuli are suppressed, and sustained focused attention is available without excessive effort. When tone is too low, signal and noise get through at similar amplitude, and sustained focus becomes genuinely impossible regardless of motivation. When tone is too high — as in states of acute stress, trauma, or chronic anxiety — the system over-selects for threat-related stimuli, and the flexible, goal-directed cognition that executive function requires becomes very difficult.

This is why atomoxetine, a selective noradrenaline reuptake inhibitor, helps some people with ADHD. It is why acute stress reliably and robustly worsens ADHD symptoms in people who are otherwise well-managed. And it is why treating ADHD in individuals with significant trauma histories, chronic anxiety, or persistently high-stress environments requires addressing the stress response — through both pharmacological and non-pharmacological means — rather than simply targeting the dopaminergic system and ignoring the noradrenergic one.

Glutamate and GABA — The Balance the Textbooks Forget

Growing research has pointed to the glutamate/GABA excitatory-inhibitory balance as a significant determinant of ADHD symptom severity and neurophysiological heterogeneity — one that is rarely discussed in standard clinical training but is directly relevant to both assessment and treatment.

Glutamate is the central nervous system's primary excitatory neurotransmitter; GABA is its primary inhibitory counterpart. Together they regulate neuronal excitability and maintain the stability of cortical networks. When this balance is disturbed toward excess excitation, the result is a brain that is too reactive, too sensitive, too easily overloaded — a profile that maps directly onto Zara's clinical presentation and onto what QEEG characterises as diffuse elevated high-beta activity.

Pathway analyses in the Demontis et al. (2019) GWAS found significant associations between glutamate-related gene sets and ADHD symptom severity, particularly hyperactivity and impulsivity. MR spectroscopy studies have documented reduced GABA concentrations in the cortex of children with ADHD, suggesting diminished inhibitory regulation. Elevated glutamate has been found in presentations overlapping with anxious, sensory-overloaded profiles — helping explain Amen's Ring of Fire subtype neurochemically.

There is a further dimension to the glutamate/GABA story that deserves attention: neuroinflammation. When microglia — the brain's immune cells — are activated by infection, prenatal stress, or chronic systemic inflammation, they release pro-inflammatory cytokines that simultaneously increase glutamate and reduce GABA activity. The excitatory accelerator goes down at the same time as the inhibitory brake is released. Studies have found elevated inflammatory markers in children with ADHD, with specific cytokines correlating with hyperactivity and inattention scores (Leffa et al., 2017; Dunn et al., 2019). Oxidative stress — a byproduct of chronic immune activation — is also consistently elevated in ADHD populations and tracks with symptom severity (Ceylan et al., 2020). This matters most where diffuse cortical overactivation, sensory hypersensitivity, and resistance to standard medications may reflect an inflammatory process actively \ sustaining the neurochemical imbalance.

The practical implication extends beyond diagnostics: the excitatory-inhibitory balance is a target for nutritional intervention in ways that the dopamine system is not. Magnesium glycinate, L-theanine, taurine, and specific B-vitamin combinations directly modulate this balance. Their evidence base is developing and, in some cases, already compelling. These interventions will be discussed in detail in Part Three.

The Three Brain Networks at the Heart of ADHD

Modern neuroscience has moved substantially beyond the model of the brain as a collection of discrete regions performing isolated functions. The current picture — emerging from decades of functional neuroimaging research — is one of large-scale dynamic networks: distributed systems of brain regions that activate together, inhibit each other, and shift in their relative dominance depending on the cognitive demands of the moment. Three networks are central to understanding both attention and its failure in ADHD.

The Default Mode Network — The Brain's Own Story

The Default Mode Network (DMN) is active during internally directed thought — self-reflection, imagination, autobiographical memory, and mind-wandering. It is the neural substrate of your inner monologue, your daydreams, your rehearsal of things you should have said differently. During tasks requiring sustained external attention, the DMN is normally suppressed. The brain turns the internal radio down so it can attend to what is outside.

In many individuals with ADHD, this suppression fails (Sonuga-Barke & Castellanos, 2007; Cortese et al., 2012). The DMN continues to fire during demanding cognitive tasks — not partially or occasionally, but persistently — competing with the Task-Positive Network for attentional resources. The result is the phenomenon every person with ADHD knows intimately and can rarely explain to people who don't have it: reading the same page three times and retaining nothing; listening to someone and suddenly realising you have been absent for the last two minutes of the conversation; sitting down to work and finding, twenty minutes later, that your mind has drifted through five entirely unrelated topics while the task has not advanced.

This is Priya's neurological experience in every lesson. Her DMN is not deficient — it is excellent. It is hyperactive at precisely the wrong moments. The effort required to continuously drag her attention back to external content is real, constant, physiologically costly, and entirely invisible from the outside — which is why she has been described as 'a pleasure to have in class' for six years while systematically not learning the material.

The Task-Positive Network — The Engine That Won't Start

The Task-Positive Network — also called the Central Executive Network — becomes active during externally directed, goal-oriented tasks. It involves the dorsolateral prefrontal cortex, the posterior parietal cortex, and associated regions responsible for working memory, planning, cognitive control, and the maintenance of task-relevant information. In healthy attention regulation, the DMN and the Task-Positive Network maintain a reciprocal, see-saw relationship: when one is active, the other is suppressed.

In ADHD, this reciprocity is disrupted. The Task-Positive Network may be chronically underactivated — making sustained effort not just unpleasant but neurologically difficult, in the same way that trying to start an engine with a weak battery is mechanically difficult. The DMN may be inadequately inhibited, constantly pulling attention inward even when external focus is required. Or, frequently, both simultaneously. The result is not laziness, not poor character, not insufficient motivation. It is a regulatory architecture that places sustained external attention significantly outside the brain's default operating range.

The Salience Network — The Broken Relevance Filter

If the DMN is the daydreamer and the Task-Positive Network is the worker, the Salience Network is the manager who decides which one gets the floor. Anchored in the anterior insula and the anterior cingulate cortex, it monitors the environment continuously for significant events and determines what deserves attentional resources. It is the brain's relevance filter.

In ADHD, the Salience Network reliably assigns excessive salience to novelty and immediate stimulation, and insufficient salience to things that are important but not immediately interesting. This is why Liam can sustain perfect, intense concentration on a skateboard trick — novel, physically immediate, providing real-time sensory feedback and social consequence — and cannot sustain attention on a maths problem that provides none of these things. The problem is not inability to concentrate. It is inability to concentrate on this, when there is a neurologically more compelling alternative available.

It also explains why medication works, at least partially: stimulants increase dopaminergic tone in precisely the circuits the Salience Network relies on, temporarily recalibrating what registers as important — making the maths problem, at least for a few hours, neurologically real in a way it wasn't before. The recalibration is temporary. The dependency on the medication to perform this function continues. But the mechanism is clear.

Figure 1: The Three Networks of the Brain in lateral and top view

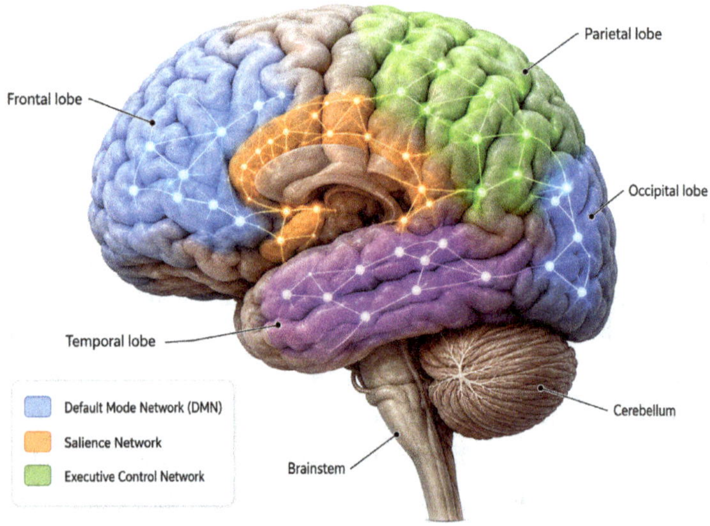

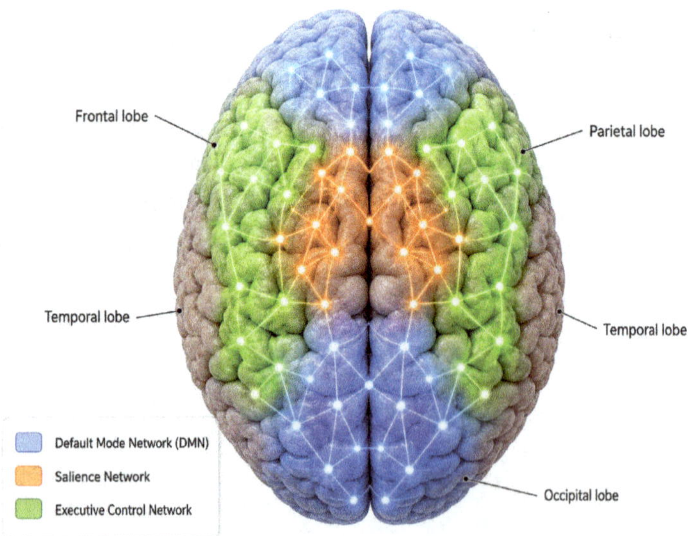

What QEEG Shows: The Electrical Fingerprint

Quantitative EEG measures the brain's electrical activity through electrodes placed on the scalp, producing maps of frequency, amplitude, and spatial distribution of brainwave activity that can be compared against normative databases drawn from age-matched individuals without neurological or psychiatric conditions. It does not produce images of brain structure. It measures brain function in real time, at millisecond resolution, in a way that MRI and CT cannot.

A brief orientation to brainwaves is helpful before going further. The brain's electrical activity is measured in frequencies — cycles per second, expressed in Hertz (Hz) — and different frequency ranges are associated with different mental states. **Delta** (1–4 Hz) is the slowest and dominates deep sleep. **Theta** (4–8 Hz) is the daydreaming frequency — associated with inattention, mind-wandering, and drowsiness when it appears during waking hours in regions that should be engaged. **Alpha** (8–12 Hz) is the brain's idling rhythm — present when the mind is relaxed and disengaged, and normally suppressed when focused attention is required. **Beta** (13–20 Hz) reflects alert, active thinking and engaged cognitive processing. **High beta** (21-40 Hz) represents states of intense cognitive or emotional activation — useful in short bursts, but associated with anxiety, sensory overload, and hypervigilance when chronically elevated. **SMR** (sensorimotor rhythm, 12–15 Hz) sits at the border of alpha and beta and is associated with calm, focused alertness and inhibitory motor control.

Figure 2: Brain Waves and their Roles

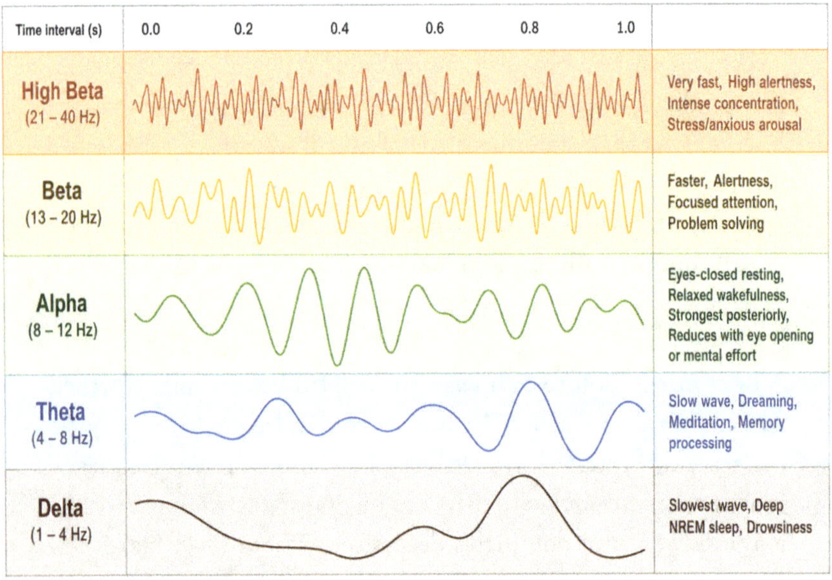

The most consistently replicated QEEG finding in ADHD is elevated theta-frequency activity (4–8 Hz) in frontal and central regions, combined with reduced beta activity (13–30 Hz) and an elevated theta/beta ratio (TBR). This pattern reflects cortical underactivation: the brain running in a slow, unfocused mode when faster, more coordinated processing is required. Think of it as an engine consistently idling when it needs to be driving.

This finding has been replicated across hundreds of studies and forms the basis of the FDA-cleared Neuropsychiatric EEG-Based Assessment Aid (NEBA) system for ADHD assessment. The theta/beta ratio also predicts treatment response: children with elevated TBR respond more strongly to methylphenidate than those without — an important clinical finding that begins to illustrate how neurophysiological profiling can guide pharmacological decisions (Arns et al., 2013).

But here is what makes QEEG so clinically important, and what the TBR-as-universal-biomarker framing systematically misses: a substantial proportion of individuals who fully meet DSM-5 criteria for ADHD do not show elevated theta or elevated TBR at all. Instead, they show patterns of elevated high-beta (20–40 Hz), excess frontal alpha, temporal dysregulation, or diffuse fast-wave activity across multiple regions. These profiles are associated with completely different clinical presentations — anxious overarousal rather than underarousal; sensory sensitivity rather than sensory-seeking; rigidity rather than distractibility; emotional volatility rather than emotional flatness — and they respond very differently to the same interventions.

Johnstone, Gunkelman, and Lunt (2005) formalised this insight in their landmark paper, proposing a framework of EEG phenotypes — stable, heritable patterns of brain electrical activity that cut across DSM categories and carry specific treatment implications. A single EEG phenotype can appear across multiple DSM diagnoses. And critically, the same DSM diagnosis can be associated with multiple distinct EEG phenotypes, each requiring a different clinical approach. Subsequent research by Arns et al. confirmed that the Frontal Slow phenotype — classic elevated theta — responds to stimulant medication, while the Slowed Alpha Peak Frequency phenotype, which can present identically on a symptom checklist, does not.

Tye, McLoughlin, Kuntsi, and Asherson (2011) established in a systematic review that QEEG measures — particularly theta power, intra-individual reaction time variability, and specific event-related potential components — meet the formal criteria for endophenotypes: they are heritable, reliably associated with ADHD, and share genetic variance with the disorder. EEG theta power heritability has been estimated at approximately 85% — among the highest heritability figures documented for any neurophysiological measure in psychiatric research. These are not soft observations. They are robust, replicable, biologically grounded findings.

The Developing Brain — A Different Timeline, Not a Fixed Ceiling

Shaw et al. (2007), using longitudinal MRI data from a large cohort of children with ADHD and typically developing controls, found that the prefrontal cortex matures an average of three years later in ADHD than in typically developing peers. This is not a subtle lag. At age seven — when school systems begin demanding sustained attention, self-regulation, and controlled impulse inhibition — the ADHD brain's primary executive regulatory system may be operating at the developmental level of a four-year-old's.

The child who cannot sit still is not defying the teacher. The child who cannot wait their turn is not choosing to be antisocial. The child who cannot sustain attention on the lesson is not being lazy. Their brain has not yet built the regulatory circuitry that would make these things possible — not because it never will, but because it is on a different developmental timeline from the one the educational system's expectations were calibrated to.

Importantly, delayed maturation is not a fixed ceiling. Developmental trajectories — unlike structural injuries — can be influenced. This is one of the neuroscientific rationales for neurophysiological training approaches: a brain that has not yet developed robust prefrontal regulation is a brain that, with the right stimulation at the right time, may develop it. The evidence for lasting effects of QEEG-guided neurofeedback — effects that persist after treatment ends, in contrast to the symptom suppression that resolves when medication is discontinued — reflects this distinction at the biological level.

In the next chapter, we turn from the brain's biology to the clinical evidence on treatment — specifically, to what the research actually shows about the long-term outcomes of current standard approaches, why some of the most important findings in this literature have received far less attention than they deserve, and what the gap between what treatment promises and what it delivers tells us about the urgency of the approach this book advocates.

References — Chapter Four

Faraone, S.V. & Larsson, H. (2019). 'Genetics of attention deficit hyperactivity disorder.' Molecular Psychiatry, 24(4), 562–575.

Demontis, D. et al. (2019). 'Discovery of the first genome-wide significant risk loci for ADHD.' Nature Genetics, 51(1), 63–75.

Pineda-Cirera, L. et al. (2019). 'Exploring genetic variation that influences brain methylation in ADHD.' Translational Psychiatry, 9, 242.

del Campo, N. et al. (2013). 'A positron emission tomography study of nigro-striatal dopaminergic mechanisms underlying attention.' Brain, 136(11), 3252–3270.

Dunn, G.A. et al. (2019). 'Neuroinflammation as a risk factor for attention deficit hyperactivity disorder.' *Pharmacology Biochemistry and Behavior*, 182, 22–34.

Leffa, D.T. et al. (2017). 'Attention-deficit/hyperactivity disorder and inflammation: what does current knowledge tell us? A systematic review.' *Frontiers in Psychiatry*, 8, 228.

Ceylan, M.F. et al. (2020). 'Role of oxidative stress and neuroinflammation in attention-deficit/hyperactivity disorder.' *Psychiatria Danubina*, 32(3–4), 399–408.

Shaw, P. et al. (2007). 'ADHD is characterized by a delay in cortical maturation.' PNAS, 104(49), 19649–19654.

Sonuga-Barke, E.J.S. & Castellanos, F.X. (2007). 'Spontaneous attentional fluctuations in impaired states.' Neuroscience & Biobehavioral Reviews, 31(7), 977–986.

Cortese, S. et al. (2012). 'Toward systems neuroscience of ADHD: a meta-analysis of 55 fMRI studies.' American Journal of Psychiatry, 169(10), 1038–1055.

Tye, C., McLoughlin, G., Kuntsi, J. & Asherson, P. (2011). 'Electrophysiological markers of genetic risk for ADHD.' Expert Reviews in Molecular Medicine, 13, e9.

Johnstone, J., Gunkelman, J. & Lunt, J. (2005). 'Clinical database development: characterization of EEG phenotypes.' Clinical EEG and Neuroscience, 36(2), 99–107.

Arns, M. et al. (2013). 'Evaluation of neurofeedback in ADHD: the long and winding road.' Biological Psychology, 95, 108–115.

Arnsten, A.F.T. (2009). 'Stress signalling pathways that impair prefrontal cortex structure and function.' Nature Reviews Neuroscience, 10(6), 410–422.

Castellanos, F.X. & Proal, E. (2012). 'Large-scale brain systems in ADHD.' Trends in Cognitive Sciences, 16(1), 17–26.

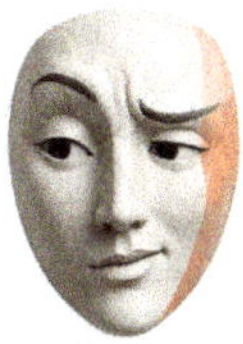

Chapter Five
The Inconvenient Follow-Up

What the evidence actually shows about long-term treatment — and why it stayed quiet

> ***DANIEL — Age 10, Thirty-Two Years Earlier:*** *The appointment is twelve minutes long. The doctor uses a Conners Parent Rating Scale and a note from Daniel's teacher. The teacher's note says he is easily distracted and struggles to complete tasks. The doctor nods. Daniel's father is given a prescription for methylphenidate. Nobody mentions that the evidence for long-term benefit is, at that point, confined to studies shorter than three months. Nobody mentions tolerance, or that the brain adapts to the drug. Nobody mentions alternatives — because in 1994, the framework for discussing alternatives has not yet been developed. The doctor has eight more patients to see before lunch. Daniel goes home with a pill and a new identity.*

There are two versions of the evidence on long-term treatment of ADHD.

The first version is the one that circulates in clinical guidelines, pharmaceutical presentations, conference symposia sponsored by medication manufacturers, and the majority of patient-facing educational materials. Stimulant medications are safe, well-tolerated, and the most rigorously studied pharmacological interventions in the history of child psychiatry. The short-term evidence is robust. Symptom scores improve in the majority of those treated. Response rates exceed those of most other psychiatric medications. The drugs are endorsed by every major clinical body in the English-speaking world and are considered the gold standard of ADHD care.

The second version is the one that emerges from the follow-up literature — the studies that tracked what happened not at fourteen months but at three years, eight years, sixteen years. It is considerably more complicated, considerably less widely disseminated, and considerably more important for anyone making long-term decisions about their own brain or their child's.

This chapter presents the second version. Not because the first is false — much of it isn't — but because the gap between what the evidence shows over time and what the clinical system communicates to patients is not a minor discrepancy. It is, in the clinical authors' assessment, a meaningful failure of informed consent. And patients deserve better.

The MTA — The Study That Reshaped Prescribing

The Multimodal Treatment Study of Children with ADHD — the MTA — is the largest, most rigorously designed, and most extensively followed clinical trial ever conducted on ADHD treatment. Funded by the US National Institute of Mental Health and conducted across six sites, it enrolled 579 children aged seven to ten with a confirmed diagnosis of combined-type ADHD and randomised them to one of four conditions: intensive medication management, intensive behavioural therapy, a combination of both, or referral to community treatment as usual.

The headline finding, published in 1999 and propagated around the world with extraordinary and lasting momentum, was unambiguous: intensive medication management was superior to behavioural therapy on core ADHD symptom measures at fourteen months. The finding was significant. It was well-powered. It was conducted with rigor. And it reshaped prescribing across the English-speaking world, providing clinical justification for medication-first approaches that have dominated ADHD care in the decades since.

The follow-up findings, published subsequently and received with considerably less fanfare, told a different story.

At twenty-four months, the advantage of medication management over behavioural therapy had reduced by approximately half. At thirty-six months, it was gone entirely. The groups that had received intensive medication management did not differ significantly from the groups that had not on any measured outcome: symptom severity, academic achievement, social functioning, or delinquency. The MTA researchers published this result: 'The modest significant advantages we found at the 24-month assessment for medication management were completely lost by 36 months' (Jensen et al., 2007, p. 998). The sixteen-year follow-up — tracking the original participants into young adulthood — found no significant differences between groups on any functional outcome: symptom severity, educational attainment, employment, relationship quality, substance use, or psychiatric hospitalisation. The most durable finding from sixteen years of follow-up was sustained suppression of height in those who had received stimulant medication.

More striking still: in some analyses of the thirty-six-month data, continued stimulant treatment was associated with higher symptom scores than discontinued treatment — suggesting that, for a proportion of children, ongoing medication was not merely failing to help but was associated with poorer outcomes than no medication. This finding was not buried in a footnote. It was published in one of the most widely read journals in child psychiatry. It received, by comparison with the original fourteen-month findings, almost no attention.

The Nieweg Analysis — When Inconvenient Findings Don't Travel

Edo Nieweg, a Dutch child psychiatrist, published a paper in 2010 in the Tijdschrift voor Psychiatrie making a point that should have been obvious but apparently required formal documentation. The MTA follow-up findings, he wrote, received 'remarkably little attention and publicity' compared to the fourteen-month results — despite being based on the same participants, the same research group, and considerably longer follow-up (Nieweg, 2010). In the Netherlands, the original 1999 finding had generated widespread adoption of medication-first treatment. The subsequent findings had generated almost nothing.

Nieweg's conclusion was direct and important: 'The dissemination of scientific knowledge is a social process.' Scientific findings do not travel on the basis of their importance or their methodological quality. They travel on the basis of whether they support or challenge existing practice, and whether they serve or undermine the interests of the institutions that fund and promote them. Knowledge that supports current prescribing practices propagates through guidelines, conferences, continuing medical education, and pharmaceutical promotional materials. Knowledge that challenges those practices requires considerably more effort to reach the clinicians and patients who need it.

This is not a conspiracy theory. It is a documented pattern, observed across multiple therapeutic areas in the peer-reviewed literature on knowledge translation, and described in detail by researchers who have no particular interest in criticising ADHD treatment specifically. The MTA is simply a particularly clear example of a general phenomenon.

The Raine Study — The Evidence That Was Excluded

The Western Australian Raine ADHD Study followed children with ADHD over years and compared long-term outcomes between those who received stimulant medication and those who did not. Its findings were broadly consistent with the MTA follow-up data: no significant differences between treated and untreated groups on core ADHD symptom scores, depression, self-perception, or social functioning at follow-up. Children treated with stimulants were, however, more likely to be rated by teachers as performing below age level on academic measures — a finding consistent with the MTA's height suppression data in suggesting that stimulant effects on ADHD symptoms may coexist with adverse effects on aspects of development that are measured less systematically (Department of Health, Western Australia, 2010).

The Raine study was not included in the 2022 AADPA Australian Evidence-Based Clinical Practice Guideline for ADHD. Bahr and Keizer's (2023) critique noted this absence pointedly: the study is Australian, locally relevant, methodologically sound, and directly contradicts the guideline's primary treatment recommendations. The guideline's stated rationale for its exclusions was not provided in the guideline document itself. Only 9% of the guideline's 134 recommendations met its own stated evidence standards. The AADPA's conference sponsors included Takeda (manufacturer of lisdexamfetamine, marketed as Vyvanse) and Novartis (manufacturer of methylphenidate, marketed as Ritalin). The guideline was funded with 1.5 million Australian dollars from the Federal Government.

This is not, it should be said, a uniquely Australian problem. The conflict-of-interest structure of guideline development in psychiatry is global, documented, and has been shown in the broader medical literature to influence the direction and strength of treatment recommendations in ways that favour the products of sponsoring manufacturers (Nejstgaard et al., 2020). Patients receiving clinical care based on these guidelines are entitled to know this.

The Side Effect Profile — What the Consent Form Should Say

The discussion of long-term efficacy failures should not proceed without an honest account of the acute and subacute side effects that accompany stimulant treatment — a profile that is well-documented in the adult literature and insufficiently communicated in most clinical encounters.

The most comprehensive analysis of methylphenidate safety in adults — a systematic review of clinical trials including 3,458 adult patients — identified the following as the most common side effects: insomnia (32%), decreased appetite (32%), headache (30%), and nervousness or anxiety (26%) (Biederman et al., 2005). These are not rare or outlying events. They affect approximately one in three adults taking the medication. In the context of ADHD subtypes, they carry particular clinical significance: insomnia worsens the attentional difficulties that medication is intended to address and compounds the neurological consequences of sleep deprivation discussed in Chapter Seventeen. Appetite suppression compromises the nutritional environment — particularly zinc, iron, and omega-3 adequacy — that is directly relevant to neurochemical function. And anxiety induction is specifically counterproductive in the Anxious and Overfocused subtypes, where stimulants may worsen the very presentation they are intended to help. The overall treatment discontinuation rate due to side effects in adults is estimated at approximately 30% — a figure rarely cited in prescriber-facing materials but representing a substantial proportion of adults initiated on stimulant treatment each year (Steer, 2005).

Mood instability and depression are among the more consequential and underacknowledged side effects in the adult population. A meta-analysis by Pozzi et al. (2018) examining emotional adverse events across paediatric and adult ADHD trials found that amphetamines specifically worsened the risk of emotional lability in a clinically meaningful proportion of patients, while methylphenidate reduced irritability and anxiety in some but increased apathy and reduced spontaneity in others. In a large nationwide population-based study from Taiwan, short-term stimulant use in ADHD patients was associated with a significantly increased probability of developing a depressive disorder compared to controls (5.3% versus 0.7%; adjusted hazard ratio 7.16, 99% CI: 6.28–8.16), raising the possibility that stimulant use may, in some individuals, precipitate or unmask depressive vulnerability (Lee et al., 2016). The rebound effect — the worsening of mood, irritability, and emotional lability that commonly occurs as a stimulant dose wears off in the late afternoon — is a clinically familiar phenomenon that is pharmacologically predictable and almost universally undertreated.

Psychosis represents the most serious psychiatric adverse effect of stimulant treatment and one that is significantly underreported in standard clinical conversations. A landmark study published in the New England Journal of Medicine by Moran et al. (2019), using a large insurance claims database of over 220,000 patients, found that new-onset psychosis occurred in 1 in 660 adolescents and young adults treated with amphetamine-based stimulants — a rate that was twice as high as with methylphenidate. The mechanism is neurobiologically coherent: amphetamines produce a more pronounced and less regulated release of dopamine than methylphenidate, and excess dopaminergic stimulation — particularly in the mesolimbic pathway — is the most well-established neurochemical substrate for psychotic symptoms. The implication is not that stimulants commonly cause psychosis — they do not — but that in individuals with personal or family history of psychosis, bipolar disorder, or significant genetic vulnerability, stimulants carry a meaningful and specific risk that should be explicitly discussed before prescription. For Ring of Fire and Anxious subtypes — where cortical overactivation and dopaminergic dysregulation are already present — this risk warrants particular vigilance.

Substance use risk is a nuanced but important consideration. The relationship between stimulant treatment and substance use disorders in adults is bidirectional and not straightforwardly harmful. Early initiation of stimulant treatment in childhood has been associated in some studies with reduced rather than increased adult substance use risk — suggesting that treated ADHD is less likely to drive self-medication through illicit substances. However, prescription stimulants themselves carry abuse and diversion potential, classified as Schedule II controlled substances precisely because of their addictive profile. In adults with active or historical substance use disorders, this risk requires explicit clinical management: extended-release formulations are preferable to immediate-release (which are more likely to be abused), non-stimulant alternatives (atomoxetine, guanfacine) should be considered as primary options, and regular clinical review of prescribing patterns is essential. The neurobiological vulnerability to stimulant misuse is not incidental; it reflects the same dopaminergic reward-pathway sensitivity that characterises ADHD itself.

Growth suppression in children, while less relevant to an adult-focused discussion, deserves mention for completeness and for the parents reading this book. Sustained stimulant treatment has been associated with reductions in final adult height of approximately one centimetre, primarily attributed to appetite suppression and its downstream effects on nutritional adequacy and growth hormone release. The MTA sixteen-year follow-up confirmed persistent height suppression in stimulant-treated participants — the most durable measurable finding from the entire study (Goldman, 2010; Molina et al., 2009).

Cardiovascular effects — consistent modest increases in heart rate (5–7 beats per minute) and blood pressure (2–4 mmHg systolic) — are well-documented across the trial literature and generally not clinically significant in healthy individuals. They carry greater implications for adults with pre-existing cardiovascular disease, hypertension, or arrhythmia. Approximately 2% of patients discontinue medication specifically due to cardiovascular adverse events, with methylphenidate associated with a 3.4% cardiovascular discontinuation rate (Storebo et al., 2017). Rare but serious events — myocardial infarction, arrhythmia, sudden cardiac death — have been reported in adults taking stimulants at standard doses, prompting FDA black box warnings for patients with known structural cardiac abnormalities.

A long-term neuroimaging study found that cumulative exposure to ADHD medication was associated with reduced hippocampal subregional volume in children — a finding that underlines the importance of minimum effective dosing and structured medication reviews rather than indefinite open-ended prescribing (Fotopoulos et al., 2021).

None of this constitutes an argument against stimulant prescribing. For the right subtype, with appropriate monitoring and realistic expectations, stimulant treatment improves function and quality of life in ways that are genuine and valuable. It is an argument for the clinical standard that should accompany any medication initiation: a frank, complete account of the side effect profile, specific to the individual's neurobiological subtype, supported by information leaflets that present the full picture rather than brushing inconvenient evidence under the carpet — and delivered in a way that gives patients the time and space to absorb what they have been told, ask questions, and return with a considered decision rather than leaving the clinic with a prescription they did not fully understand. Informed consent is not a signature on a form. It is a process. And for a Schedule II controlled substance prescribed to a developing brain or a vulnerable adult, that process deserves the seriousness it has too rarely been given.

Diversion — The Risk Nobody Talks About at the School Gate

Stimulant medications prescribed for ADHD are classified as Schedule II controlled substances — the same regulatory category as opioids like morphine and codeine — because they carry a documented and significant potential for abuse, dependence, and diversion. This is not a bureaucratic technicality. It is a pharmacological reality that the cultural normalisation of ADHD medication has quietly eroded from public consciousness.

Diversion — the transfer of a prescribed controlled substance to someone for whom it was not prescribed — is more common in the ADHD context than most people who engage in it recognise as a problem. It takes forms that feel entirely benign: noticing a friend struggling to concentrate before an exam and offering them one of your tablets. Letting a partner try your medication because they suspect they might have ADHD too. Accepting a colleague's Ritalin for a difficult afternoon because yours has worn off. These gestures feel like helpfulness. They are, in law, a criminal offence — and more importantly, they are a genuine clinical risk.

Stimulants are not universally safe. As this chapter has documented, they carry real risks of elevated blood pressure, cardiac arrhythmia, anxiety, psychosis, and mood instability — risks that are managed in a clinical context through history-taking, subtype assessment, comorbidity screening, and ongoing monitoring. None of that protective infrastructure exists when a tablet is shared over a kitchen table. The person receiving it has no established diagnosis, no cardiovascular risk evaluation, and no prescriber who will follow up. If they have an unrecognised Ring of Fire or Anxious ADHD profile, the stimulant they have just taken may worsen their condition significantly. If they have a contraindication to stimulants, the consequences could be considerably more serious.

It is worth being direct: sharing a stimulant prescription is not meaningfully different from sharing any other recreational substance. The fact that one person's name is on the bottle does not make the act of passing it to someone else less of a diversion. It is, in effect, the respectable face of recreational stimulant use — which is precisely why Schedule II classification exists, and precisely why the cultural tendency to treat ADHD medication as a productivity tool rather than a controlled drug requires consistent clinical pushback.

If someone in your life is struggling with attention, concentration, or executive function, the appropriate response is to encourage them toward proper assessment — not to offer them a shortcut that bypasses the process designed to keep them safe.

Tolerance — The Phenomenon That Guidelines Refuse to Discuss

Tolerance to a pharmacological agent — the progressive reduction of its effects with continued use, requiring dose escalation to maintain the original response — is well-understood pharmacology across most drug classes. In ADHD pharmacology, it receives remarkably little systematic clinical attention despite being well-documented in the literature.

Handelman and Sumiya (2022), reviewing the published evidence on stimulant tolerance in ADHD, found two distinct patterns. Early tolerance — loss of therapeutic response within days or weeks of initiation — was documented in 24.7% of patients in a retrospective chart review, all receiving doses in or above the upper therapeutic range. Gradual tolerance — slow attenuation of response over months and years — is suggested by the MTA data (66% of children showing waning benefit by thirty-six months) and by a meta-regression of forty-four adult ADHD medication trials, which found that longer study duration predicted smaller effect sizes across the range studied (4–26 weeks), consistent with progressive pharmacodynamic adaptation (Cunill et al., 2016).

The biological mechanism is documented and coherent. Chronic methylphenidate administration in animal models produces upregulation of the dopamine transporter and increased autoreceptor sensitivity — adaptive changes in the precise molecular machinery the drug acts on, which progressively reduce its net effect. Wang et al. (2013) documented a 24% increase in striatal dopamine transporter availability in adults taking methylphenidate for twelve months — a measured neurobiological change demonstrating that pharmacodynamic adaptation is occurring even in patients whose clinical questionnaire scores suggest continued response. The drug is working against increasingly robust molecular resistance. This resistance does not appear on a symptom rating scale until it has already become substantial.

Handelman and Sumiya reviewed published clinical guidelines from the United States, Europe, Canada, and Germany for guidance on tolerance management. Only the Canadian guidelines mentioned the concept. None provided specific clinical guidance on how to identify it or what to do when it occurs. In a field where a significant proportion of long-term patients appear to be experiencing gradual loss of benefit, this represents a meaningful gap in the clinical guidance infrastructure — one whose practical consequences fall not on the guidelines but on the patients.

What Amphetamine Does to the Brain Over Time

Beyond pharmacological tolerance, a growing body of neurobiological research has examined what happens to brain structure and function with long-term stimulant exposure. Berman, Kuczenski, McCracken, and London's (2009) comprehensive review in Molecular Psychiatry noted that effects of prolonged stimulant treatment 'have not been fully explored' and that understanding such effects 'is a research priority' — a priority that, more than fifteen years later, remains substantially unmet.

What animal models show is consistent and should be communicated clearly to patients: chronic amphetamine administration produces changes in dopaminergic terminal morphology, alterations in receptor density, signs of oxidative stress in affected brain regions, and adaptive changes in multiple molecular systems. Whether therapeutic doses in humans produce comparable changes over extended periods is not definitively established — because the necessary long-term controlled human studies have not been conducted. This is not evidence of safety.

It is an absence of evidence in one direction, in a context where there is substantial evidence of neurobiological effects in another.

Basmadjian et al. (2021), examining the effects of repeated amphetamine administration in an animal model, found acute oxidative stress, long-lasting glial reactivity persisting twenty-one days after the last dose, and transient angiogenesis — all in the prefrontal cortex, the brain region most critical for the executive function deficits that ADHD treatment targets. These findings require cautious extrapolation to clinical populations. But they provide a documented biological mechanism through which long-term amphetamine exposure might produce lasting structural and functional changes in precisely the cortical region that matters most — changes invisible on structural MRI but potentially detectable, and perhaps reversible, through the functional lens of QEEG.

Berman et al. (2009) documented that amphetamine-induced psychosis — clinically indistinguishable from acute schizophrenia — has been observed in individuals receiving prescription doses, not only in recreational users. In a controlled study cited in their review, repeated oral dextroamphetamine produced full paranoid psychosis in all four healthy volunteers who participated, at cumulative doses of 120 to 750 milligrams — doses achievable, in a patient receiving a standard adult therapeutic dose of 30 milligrams per day, over a period of four to twenty-five days. This finding is not an argument that stimulant medications should not be prescribed. It is an argument that their prescription should be guided by more than a symptom rating scale, calibrated to the specific brain receiving them, and monitored over time with the rigour that a Schedule II controlled substance with this pharmacological profile warrants.

The Thirty-Year Follow-Up — What Long-Term Outcomes Actually Show

Satterfield et al. (2007) reported thirty-year prospective follow-up data on 254 white hyperactive boys from Los Angeles, followed from childhood (age 6–12) to mid-adulthood (age 18–38) using official California state arrest records. The results were sobering: hyperactive boys had significantly higher rates of arrest (44%), conviction (29%), and incarceration (26%) compared to non-hyperactive controls. The findings were not unexpected given what is known about ADHD and externalising behaviour.

What was clinically important was the treatment comparison. Boys who had received intensive three-year multimodality treatment — combining medication with years of psychological, educational, and family intervention — did not differ significantly from boys who had received medication alone on adult criminal outcomes. Neither treatment approach was protective against adult criminality in this high-risk subsample.

This finding should not be read as an argument that treatment doesn't matter. It is an argument that treatments which target only the surface symptoms — without addressing the underlying neurobiological heterogeneity, the co-occurring conditions, the nutritional vulnerabilities, and the environmental determinants of risk — are insufficient for the goals we have set for ADHD treatment. The symptom-suppressing functions of stimulant medication are real and often valuable. The claim that symptom suppression over months or years translates into improved adult functional outcomes is substantially less well-supported than the clinical consensus suggests.

What This Evidence Means for Clinical Practice

Let us be clear about what this chapter is and is not. It is not a manifesto against medication. It is not a brief for the anti-psychiatry movement. It is not an invitation to stop treatment, distrust prescribers, or seek validation for a decision already made. It is something considerably more demanding than any of those things: an honest account of what the evidence actually shows, written for people who deserve to make decisions about their own brains — or their children's brains — with full information rather than curated reassurance.

There is a force working against that honesty that deserves naming directly. Social media has generated an extraordinary volume of ADHD content — much of it created by people who are neither clinicians nor researchers, speaking with a confidence that their credentials do not support. The ADHD community online is, in many respects, a remarkable thing: validating, connecting, and destigmatising in ways that formal medicine has consistently failed to achieve. But it has also created a cultural pressure — felt acutely by prescribers — in which medication is celebrated as liberation, side effects are minimised as the price of functioning, and any clinical hesitation is reframed as ignorance or gatekeeping. It is thus important to point out that the enthusiasm of the well-intentioned is not a substitute for the judgment of the well-informed.

What this chapter argues for, then, is precision, honesty, and the courage to hold the full picture. It argues for telling patients that the short-term evidence for stimulant efficacy is strong, and that the long-term evidence for functional benefit is considerably weaker than guideline recommendations imply. It argues for monitoring tolerance systematically rather than attributing waning response to inadequate dosing. It argues for treating the neurobiological consequences of long-term amphetamine exposure as a genuine clinical consideration rather than a theoretical footnote. And it argues, most fundamentally, for using the tools that are now available — including QEEG and continuous performance testing, the subjects of Part Two — to understand the specific brain before selecting and monitoring the treatment. The label got us this far. The brain will take us the rest of the way.

References — Chapter Five

Jensen, P.S. et al. (2007). '3-year follow-up of the NIMH MTA study.' Journal of the American Academy of Child & Adolescent Psychiatry, 46(8), 989–1002.

Molina, B.S.G. et al. (2009). 'The MTA at 8 years: prospective follow-up of children treated for combined-type ADHD.' Journal of the American Academy of Child & Adolescent Psychiatry, 48(5), 484–500.

Swanson, J.M. et al. (2017). 'Young adult outcomes in the follow-up of the MTA study.' Journal of Child Psychology and Psychiatry, 58(6), 663–678.

Nieweg, E.H. (2010). 'Is ADHD-medicatie na 2–3 jaar uitgewerkt? Over de verrassende, maar weinig bekende follow-up van het MTA-onderzoek.' Tijdschrift voor Psychiatrie, 52(4), 245–253.

Department of Health, Western Australia. (2010). Raine ADHD Study: Long-term outcomes associated with stimulant medication in the treatment of ADHD in children. Perth: Government of Western Australia.

Bahr, G. & Keizer, J. (2023). 'When guidelines fail: fundamental problems with the AADPA guideline for ADHD.' Journal of the New Zealand College of Clinical Psychologists, 33(1), 45–55.

Handelman, K. & Sumiya, F. (2022). 'Tolerance to stimulant medication for attention deficit hyperactivity disorder: literature review and case report.' Brain Sciences, 12(8), 959.

Cunill, R. et al. (2016). 'Efficacy, safety and variability in pharmacotherapy for adults with ADHD: a meta-analysis.' Psychopharmacology, 233(1), 187–197.

Wang, G.J. et al. (2013). 'Long-term stimulant treatment affects brain dopamine transporter level in patients with ADHD.' PLoS ONE, 8(5), e63023.

Berman, S.M., Kuczenski, R., McCracken, J.T. & London, E.D. (2009). 'Potential adverse effects of amphetamine treatment on brain and behavior: a review.' Molecular Psychiatry, 14(2), 123–142.

Basmadjian, O.M. et al. (2021). 'Amphetamine induces oxidative stress, glial activation and transient angiogenesis in prefrontal cortex via AT1-R.' Frontiers in Pharmacology, 12, 647747.

Nejstgaard, C.H. et al. (2020). 'Conflicts of interest in clinical guidelines, advisory committee reports, opinion pieces, and narrative reviews.' Cochrane Database of Systematic Reviews, 12, MR000040.

Biederman, J., Spencer, T. & Wilens, T. (2005). 'Evidence-based pharmacotherapy for attention-deficit hyperactivity disorder.' *International Journal of Neuropsychopharmacology*, 7(1), 77–97.

Steer, C. (2005). 'Managing attention deficit/hyperactivity disorder: unmet needs and future directions.' *Archives of Disease in Childhood*, 90(Suppl 1), i19–25.

Moran, L.V. et al. (2019). 'Psychosis with methylphenidate or amphetamine in patients with ADHD.' *New England Journal of Medicine*, 380(12), 1128–1138.

Pozzi, M. et al. (2018). 'Adverse drug events related to mood and emotion in paediatric patients treated for ADHD: a meta-analysis.' *Journal of Affective Disorders*, 238, 161–178.

Lee, M.J. et al. (2016). 'Attention-deficit hyperactivity disorder, its treatment with medication and the probability of developing a depressive disorder: a nationwide population-based study in Taiwan.' *Journal of Affective Disorders*, 189, 110–117.

Storebo, O.J. et al. (2017). 'Cardiovascular effects of stimulant and non-stimulant medication for children and adolescents with ADHD.' *CNS Drugs*, 31(3), 199–211.

Fotopoulos, N.H. et al. (2021). 'Cumulative exposure to ADHD medication is inversely related to hippocampus subregional volume in children.' *NeuroImage: Clinical*, 31, 102695.

Goldman, R.D. (2010). 'ADHD stimulants and their effect on height in children.' *Canadian Family Physician*, 56(2), 145–146.

Krinzinger, H. et al. (2019). 'Neurological and psychiatric adverse effects of long-term methylphenidate treatment in ADHD: a map of the current evidence.' *Neuroscience & Biobehavioral Reviews*, 107, 945–968.

Satterfield, J.H. et al. (2007). 'A 30-year prospective follow-up study of hyperactive boys with conduct problems.' Journal of the American Academy of Child & Adolescent Psychiatry, 46(5), 601–610.

Insel, T. (2013). 'Transforming diagnosis.' Director's Blog, National Institute of Mental Health.

PART TWO
Seeing the Brain Behind the Label

Part One established the problem: a diagnostic system that is descriptively useful and aetiologically uninformative, applied to a condition that is neurobiologically heterogeneous, producing treatments that are selected by category rather than by biology. If ADHD were a single, uniform condition with a single mechanism, this would be acceptable clinical practice. It is not. The same behavioural label covers meaningfully different brains — and different brains require different approaches.

Part Two is the turn from problem to solution. It begins with the tools: the objective measures that move assessment beyond symptom observation into the territory of neurophysiology, and the brain-imaging approaches that make the invisible architecture of attention visible. It then devotes a full chapter to each of the seven major neurobiological subtypes of ADHD — not the three DSM presentations, but the seven brain patterns that clinical and neurophysiological research has consistently identified as meaningfully distinct.

For each subtype, we examine the symptom cluster, the brain imaging correlates, the neurochemical profile, the conditions it is commonly confused with and how to distinguish between them, and the specific treatment implications — for medication, supplements, and neurofeedback. Throughout, our seven characters continue their journeys, with more hope than before.

The goal of Part Two is not to provide a diagnostic manual. It is to show what becomes possible when we treat the brain rather than the label — and to make the case, through seven specific examples, for why that distinction matters in clinical practice.

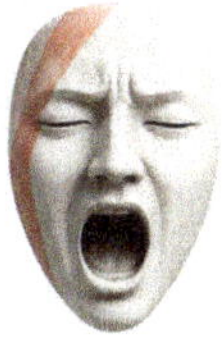

Chapter Six

Beyond the Checklist

Rating scales, IQ tests, CPTs, SPECT, and QEEG — what each can and cannot tell you

> ***ALL SEVEN — Present Day:*** *Liam is 25 and awaiting sentencing. Priya is 27 and has been on her second antidepressant for eight months with partial response. Oliver is 34 and seeing a couples therapist who has suggested the problem might be his rigidity. Zara is 28 and has just been told by a psychiatrist that she is 'treatment resistant.' Daniel is 42 and has started his fourth career. Maya is 38 and has recently been promoted and is convinced there has been an administrative error. Amir is 32 and has been treated for anxiety for four years while the attention difficulties that drive it go unaddressed. All seven have had assessments. None has had a brain assessment. This is about to change.*

There is a thought experiment that deserves wider currency in clinical psychiatry.

Imagine that a cardiologist's assessment of a patient with chest pain consisted of asking the patient to rate the severity of their symptoms on a scale of one to ten, having their family members complete a questionnaire about how breathless they seem, and reviewing their school records to see if they had ever complained of feeling tired. No ECG. No echocardiogram. No stress test. No imaging. Just the symptoms, rated by the people observing them.

We would not consider this cardiology. We would consider it dangerously inadequate. And yet this is, with only modest exaggeration, the standard of objective measurement applied to ADHD assessment in most clinical settings. The question this chapter asks is straightforward: what objective tools exist for ADHD assessment, what do they actually measure, and why — given all of this — is QEEG not already the standard of care?

The Rating Scale: Useful, Biased, and Widely Overvalued

Rating scales — the Conners, the ADHD Rating Scale, the Brown Executive Function Scales, the Vanderbilt, and their various iterations — are the workhorses of ADHD assessment. They are quick, inexpensive, reproducible, and familiar to clinicians across settings. They are also, when used as the primary or sole basis for diagnosis, fundamentally inadequate.

The problem is not that rating scales measure nothing. They measure something real: the frequency and severity of specific behaviours as observed and reported by specific people in specific contexts. The problem is that what they measure is not what we need to know.

First, they are profoundly subject to rater bias. A teacher who finds a child's energy exhausting will rate them differently from a teacher who finds that same energy charming. A parent in a crisis household will rate their child's symptoms more severely than the same parent in a period of stability. A child assessed during a difficult term will look more symptomatic than the same child assessed during the summer holidays. None of this reflects anything about the child's brain.

Second, they are non-specific. As established in Part One, the core ADHD symptom clusters — inattention, impulsivity, restlessness — appear in anxiety disorders, depression, sleep disorders, thyroid dysfunction, iron deficiency, trauma responses, and giftedness in understimulating environments. A rating scale that scores 'above threshold' tells you that the person is experiencing clinically significant attentional difficulty. It tells you nothing about why.

Third, they are subject to systematic demographic biases. Girls consistently score lower than boys on hyperactive-impulsive items, resulting in later diagnosis despite equivalent or greater impairment. Younger children in school year cohorts score higher, producing the relative age effect documented across multiple national datasets. Children from different cultural backgrounds are rated differently by teachers from the majority culture. These are not minor measurement artefacts. They are structural failures of the assessment tool.

Fourth — and most critically for the phenotypic approach this book advocates — they cannot distinguish between neurophysiological subtypes. A child with classic ADHD (frontal theta excess, dopaminergic underactivation) and a child with Ring of Fire ADHD (diffuse cortical overactivation, glutamatergic dysregulation) will produce statistically similar profiles on a Conners rating scale. The identical scores will, in the standard clinical pathway, lead to the identical treatment. In the Ring of Fire child, that treatment will commonly make things worse.

The IQ Test: What It Measures — and Why ADHD Assessments Shouldn't Stop There

The Wechsler Adult Intelligence Scale (WAIS) and its predecessors and derivatives are among the most widely administered instruments in psychological assessment. They are sophisticated, well-normed, extensively validated tools for measuring intellectual ability across multiple domains. They are also, in the context of ADHD assessment specifically, often used to answer a question they were not designed to answer.

The rationale for including comprehensive intelligence testing in ADHD assessments is defensible: ADHD is associated with variability in cognitive performance across domains; specific learning disabilities that require differential diagnosis co-occur frequently with ADHD; and some patterns of cognitive performance — notably the Working Memory Index and Processing Speed Index of the WAIS — are frequently lower in ADHD than the other indices, producing a characteristic profile. This profile is clinically informative.

What it is not is diagnostically specific. The same patterns — reduced working memory performance, slow processing speed, variable performance across domains — appear in anxiety, depression, sleep disorders, and multiple other conditions. A dissociated WAIS profile in the direction associated with ADHD does not confirm ADHD. A normal WAIS profile does not exclude it. Many highly intelligent individuals with ADHD — including Oliver in our cast of seven — score uniformly in the superior range on all indices, because their intelligence compensates for their executive function difficulties in precisely the structured, time-limited, one-on-one testing environment that IQ assessment provides.

This is one of the most common failure modes in ADHD assessment. The psychologist concludes: 'This individual's cognitive profile does not support a diagnosis of ADHD,' because the test scores are even and high. What they are observing is compensation, not absence of disorder. Oliver's ADHD is most visible not in a structured testing room with a sympathetic examiner and no competing stimuli, but in the open-plan office with seventeen emails, an upcoming deadline, and his colleague asking him about last night's meeting at the moment he was in the middle of a completely different thought.

IQ testing is valuable. In ADHD assessment, it should be understood as one piece of a larger picture — informative about intellectual strengths and some specific cognitive difficulties, but neither sufficient nor specific enough to carry diagnostic weight on its own.

Continuous Performance Tests: The First Move Toward Objectivity

Continuous Performance Tests (CPTs) represent a genuinely significant step toward objective ADHD assessment. Rather than relying on what others report about behaviour, they measure attention and impulse control directly, under standardised conditions, using computerised paradigms that are reproducible across assessors and settings.

The basic paradigm is elegant in its simplicity: the individual sits at a computer and responds (or withholds response) to a series of stimuli presented at set intervals over a sustained period, typically fifteen to twenty-two minutes. The computer measures, precisely, how often they correctly respond to target stimuli (hits), how often they fail to respond when they should (omissions, measuring inattention), how often they respond when they shouldn't (commissions, measuring impulsivity), and how variable their response speed is across the task (reaction time variability, measuring inconsistent attention). These measures are then compared against a normative database of age- and sex-matched individuals without ADHD.

The resulting profile is considerably more objective than any rating scale, immune to rater bias, standardised across administrations, and sensitive to the specific attentional and inhibitory dimensions that are neurologically most characteristic of ADHD. Two CPTs have accumulated the most robust evidence bases and the strongest clinical track records.

The TOVA — Test of Variables of Attention

The TOVA (Test of Variables of Attention) is a non-language-based CPT that uses simple geometric figures as stimuli, deliberately avoiding letters and numbers to eliminate the influence of reading ability and educational history on performance. Participants respond to a target figure and withhold response to a non-target, across a 21.6-minute administration. The test is divided into two halves with deliberately different target frequencies — the first half has infrequent targets (testing vigilance), the second has frequent targets (testing inhibition) — allowing assessment of how performance varies across different attentional demands.

The TOVA generates four primary variables: response time (processing speed), response time variability (consistency of attention), commission errors (impulsivity), and omission errors (inattention). These are expressed as standard scores relative to the normative database, with a composite ADHD score. Sensitivity for ADHD ranges from approximately 72–87% depending on the population studied and the threshold applied; specificity ranges from approximately 73–85% (Greenberg & Waldman,

1993; Leark et al., 1996). The TOVA is also used to monitor medication response — the same standardised measurement taken before and after medication initiation provides objective evidence of treatment effect on attentional performance, independent of parent or teacher report.

One important and frequently underappreciated feature of the TOVA is its sensitivity to ADHD in the inattentive presentation specifically — a population that, because of reduced hyperactivity and impulsivity, is frequently underidentified on behavioural measures. Omission errors and elevated response time variability in the first (low-frequency) half of the test are particularly characteristic of this presentation, and can identify individuals whose quiet, non-disruptive presentation has passed under the clinical radar for years. For Priya, the TOVA is likely to be the first objective test in her life that returns an unambiguously positive result.

The IVA — Integrated Visual and Auditory CPT

The IVA (Integrated Visual and Auditory Continuous Performance Test) adds an important dimension to the CPT approach: it assesses attentional and inhibitory performance across both visual and auditory modalities simultaneously. Stimuli — the numbers 1 and 2 — are presented in alternating visual and auditory form, and the participant must respond to targets and withhold responses to non-targets across both channels over a 13-minute administration.

The IVA produces twelve primary scales organised into two composite quotients: the Response Control Quotient (measuring impulsivity in both visual and auditory domains) and the Attention Quotient (measuring inattention in both domains). This dual-modality design allows detection of modality-specific attentional differences — some individuals show greater difficulty in the auditory than the visual domain, or vice versa — a finding that has implications for educational and environmental accommodations as well as for understanding the neurological profile.

Sensitivity for the IVA ranges from approximately 80–90%; specificity from 75–88% (Tinius, 2003). Like the TOVA, it has an established track record in medication monitoring and is particularly useful in longitudinal assessment — when administered at regular intervals, it provides an objective index of whether attentional performance is improving, stable, or declining. In the context of the tolerance concerns discussed in Chapter Five, regular TOVA or IVA administration provides one of the few objective ways to detect waning medication effect before it becomes clinically apparent through symptom return.

What CPTs Can — and Cannot — Tell You

CPTs represent a meaningful advance over rating scales. They are objective, standardised, modality-specific, sensitive to the specific attentional and inhibitory dimensions most relevant to ADHD, and capable of detecting presentations that behavioural observation misses. In combination with clinical interview and developmental history, they add genuine diagnostic value.

They also have limitations that are important to communicate clearly, and that directly motivate the integration with QEEG that this chapter is building toward.

What CPTs Cannot Measure: Executive Function

ADHD's impairment is not limited to attention and impulse control in the narrow sense that CPTs measure. Executive function — the constellation of higher-order cognitive processes that includes planning, cognitive flexibility, working memory, inhibitory control in real-world contexts, and self-monitoring — is among the most characteristic and consequential domains of difficulty in ADHD. And it is precisely the domain that CPTs assess most poorly.

This is partly a problem of ecological validity: the CPT is a highly structured, repetitive, single-task paradigm with no competing stimuli, clear rules, and immediate feedback. Executive function difficulties in ADHD are most pronounced in open-ended, multi-step, competing-demand environments — the office, the classroom, the kitchen at 6 p.m. with three things happening simultaneously. The same cognitive systems that fail in these environments may perform adequately in the constrained, predictable CPT context. The test is measuring attention under conditions optimised for attention; it is not measuring executive function under conditions that tax it.

One tool designed specifically to address the executive function gap in CPT-based assessment is the MeSA (Metacognitive and Executive Skills Assessment), developed as a companion to the IVA-2. Where the IVA-2 measures attention and impulse control under standardised conditions, the MeSA extends the assessment into the domains of attention control and cognitive flexibility — two core components of executive function that CPTs alone do not capture. It is designed to be interpreted alongside the IVA-2 report, allowing the clinician to compare attentional performance with executive control strengths and weaknesses in the same individual. It is best understood at this stage as a clinically useful adjunct — one that meaningfully extends the scope of objective assessment beyond what CPTs provide — rather than an independently validated diagnostic tool in its own right.

What CPTs Cannot Measure: Emotional Dysregulation

As established in Chapter Two, emotional dysregulation is present in up to 70% of adults with ADHD, may account for more functional impairment than the core attentional symptoms, and is entirely absent from the DSM criteria. It is also entirely absent from CPT assessment. A person with severe rejection sensitive dysphoria, chronic emotional volatility, and catastrophic responses to minor failure will produce a CPT profile identical to a person whose ADHD is characterised almost entirely by cognitive attentional difficulties with minimal emotional component. The CPT cannot distinguish between them — and because the distinction is clinically important for treatment selection, its absence from standard assessment represents a meaningful gap.

The Hyperfocus Problem

Perhaps the most clinically significant limitation of CPTs — and one that produces systematic false negatives in a diagnostically important population — is their vulnerability to hyperfocus. The CPT paradigm, particularly for individuals who find computerised tasks inherently engaging or who are motivated to perform well on an assessment, can inadvertently trigger hyperfocus: the state of sustained, absorbed attention that many people with ADHD can achieve when a task provides sufficient novelty, stakes, or stimulation.

An adult with ADHD who is motivated during the assessment— or who finds the computerised format intrinsically engaging — may perform in the normal or superior range. Their ADHD does not disappear during the test; it is temporarily suppressed by a level of cognitive engagement that does not generalise to the rest of their functioning. Clinicians who rely primarily on CPT results may incorrectly conclude that the presentation is not consistent with ADHD, when in fact it is consistent with a profile of ADHD in which motivation and novelty can temporarily override the attentional deficit. This is most likely to occur in high-intelligence individuals — Oliver, for example, would be at significant risk of a false-negative CPT result — and in individuals with the overfocused or anxious subtypes, who tend to hyperfocus under evaluative pressure.

The solution is not to abandon CPTs but to interpret them within a broader assessment framework — one that includes not just what the person can do under optimal conditions but what their brain is doing neurophysiologically at rest and during cognitive challenge.

SPECT Imaging — The Brain in Three Dimensions

Single Photon Emission Computed Tomography (SPECT) produces three-dimensional maps of cerebral blood flow — a proxy for regional brain activity — by tracking the distribution of a radioactive tracer injected intravenously. Unlike MRI, which produces static structural images, SPECT captures brain function: which regions are active, which are underactive, and how the pattern of activity changes between rest and cognitive challenge.

Daniel Amen's clinical research programme, spanning decades and encompassing one of the largest private brain SPECT databases in the world, has made the case that different presentations of ADHD are characterised by distinguishable SPECT patterns — and that these patterns have direct implications for medication selection and treatment planning. His typology, which forms the basis for much of the subtype framework in this book, identifies patterns including prefrontal hypoperfusion (Classic and Inattentive ADHD), anterior cingulate hyperperfusion (Overfocused), temporal lobe abnormalities (Temporal Lobe type), limbic hyperactivation (Limbic type), and diffuse cortical overactivation (Ring of Fire) — each correlating with distinct clinical presentations and treatment responses (Amen, 2013).

The clinical value of SPECT in ADHD assessment is substantial. It provides a three-dimensional, functionally dynamic view of the brain that neither structural MRI nor CPTs can offer. It has been used to demonstrate that stimulant medications help some ADHD presentations while worsening others — a finding visible in blood flow changes that provides objective biological grounding for what clinicians have observed empirically but struggled to predict systematically.

Its limitations, however, are also substantial and are important to acknowledge honestly.

SPECT involves exposure to ionising radiation — not a trivial consideration when the indication is a neurodevelopmental condition rather than cancer staging, and particularly not trivial when the patient is a child or an individual who may require repeated assessments. The radiation dose from a clinical SPECT scan is modest by medical imaging standards but is not zero, and repeated imaging carries cumulative risk.

SPECT is expensive. A clinical SPECT study costs considerably more than most psychiatric assessment tools. It requires specialised equipment available only at a small number of centres globally. It is not covered by most insurance systems for ADHD assessment. And it requires intravenous injection, which is neither comfortable nor universally acceptable, and which introduces a procedural element that can affect the performance of anxious individuals.

Finally, SPECT resolution is limited compared to fMRI and does not capture the millisecond-by-millisecond dynamics of neural network activity that electroencephalography provides. Blood flow changes lag neural activity by seconds; SPECT captures a relatively coarse temporal window of brain function rather than the real-time dynamics that determine attentional performance.

QEEG — The Office-Based, Radiation-Free Brain Map

Quantitative EEG, introduced in Chapter Four, deserves its own extended treatment here in the context of why it is clinically preferable to SPECT for routine ADHD assessment — not because SPECT data is uninformative (it is very informative), but because QEEG provides comparable clinical utility at a fraction of the cost, without radiation, without injection, without specialist centre access, and with considerably greater temporal resolution.

The practical procedure is simple enough to describe in a clinical leaflet. The patient sits comfortably in a chair in the clinician's office. A cap embedded with nineteen or more electrodes is placed on the scalp, with conductive gel applied to ensure good signal contact. The patient is asked to sit quietly, sometimes with eyes open and sometimes closed, for approximately twenty minutes. They may also perform a brief cognitive task while recording continues. No injections. No radioactive tracers. No specialised imaging suite. The data is collected, processed by QEEG analysis software, and compared against a normative database of age-matched individuals — producing maps of frequency band power, coherence, and phase across the cortex that are directly interpretable in clinical terms.

The QEEG provides information that SPECT does not, and vice versa. SPECT shows blood flow distribution — a metabolic proxy for sustained regional activity. QEEG shows electrical oscillation patterns — the direct product of neuronal communication, with millisecond temporal resolution. They are complementary rather than competitive. Where SPECT excels is in visualising the three-dimensional distribution of functional activity across the whole brain, including subcortical structures that EEG cannot reach. Where QEEG excels is in capturing the dynamic, oscillatory nature of cortical activity that underlies moment-to-moment attentional regulation — precisely the biological substrate of attention and its disorders.

For most clinical purposes — initial ADHD subtype identification, neurofeedback protocol design, monitoring of treatment response, and longitudinal tracking of brain function change — QEEG provides the relevant information at accessible cost and without the risks associated with ionising radiation. Where the clinical picture is complex, ambiguous, or involves suspected subcortical pathology, SPECT remains a valuable adjunct. In most routine clinical presentations, QEEG is the appropriate starting point.

Combining CPTs and QEEG: The Sum Greater Than Its Parts

The most informative assessment approach combines objective behavioural measurement (CPT) with direct neurophysiological measurement (QEEG), interpreted alongside detailed clinical history, developmental assessment, and collateral information.

CPTs contribute information about attentional and inhibitory performance under standardised conditions: how accurately, how consistently, and how quickly the person responds across sustained attentional demand, in both visual and auditory modalities. QEEG contributes information about the neurophysiological substrate of those performances: what the brain's electrical activity looks like at rest and during cognitive challenge, which frequency patterns dominate, which regions show abnormal activity, and — crucially — which neurophysiological phenotype the brain most closely corresponds to.

Together, they answer different versions of the same question. The CPT asks: how well does this brain perform on attentional tasks? The QEEG asks: why? The CPT tells you the functional outcome. The QEEG tells you the biological mechanism. And the biological mechanism, as the subtype chapters that follow will demonstrate, determines which treatment is indicated, which medication profile is likely to help or harm, which neurofeedback protocol is appropriate, and which nutritional or functional interventions are most likely to be beneficial.

A TOVA or IVA result showing impaired attention and elevated impulsivity, combined with a QEEG showing elevated frontal theta, strongly implicates Classic ADHD and indicates a dopaminergic treatment target. The same CPT result combined with a QEEG showing diffuse elevated high-beta implicates Ring of Fire ADHD and contra-indicates stimulant medication. The same behavioural performance, interpreted through completely different neurophysiology, leading to completely different treatment decisions. This is the clinical case for the combined assessment model.

In the chapters that follow, we will examine each of the seven major neurobiological ADHD subtypes in turn — using exactly this combined framework to illuminate what makes each type distinct, how each is commonly confused with other conditions, and what the specific neurophysiology tells us about the best treatment approach.

A Note on BCIA Accreditation and Neurofeedback Protocols

Throughout the subtype chapters, we will describe the neurofeedback protocols most commonly associated with each neurophysiological profile. A crucial caveat accompanies all of these descriptions, and it bears stating clearly at the outset.

Neurofeedback protocols are not static prescriptions. They are starting points that must be continuously adapted as the brain responds to training. As the brain reorganises — as previously underactivated circuits begin to function, as excess slow waves reduce, as inter-regional coherence patterns normalise — the appropriate training targets change. A protocol that is optimal in week two may be counterproductive in week twelve. The brain is not a machine to be programmed; it is a living system that adapts. Effective neurofeedback requires a practitioner who can read the QEEG, interpret the ongoing changes in the brain's electrical landscape, and adjust the protocol accordingly — not one who applies the same protocol to every person who walks through the door.

For this reason, we strongly recommend that neurofeedback be delivered by a clinician holding BCIA (Biofeedback Certification International Alliance) accreditation in neurofeedback, who is also trained and experienced in QEEG interpretation. BCIA accreditation requires completion of an approved didactic training programme, a supervised clinical internship, and passage of a written examination — providing a minimum standard of competence. QEEG-guided neurofeedback — where protocol design is based on the individual's specific brain electrical profile rather than on DSM diagnosis or behavioural presentation alone — has been demonstrated to produce superior outcomes compared to behaviourally guided approaches (Johnstone et al., 2005). The protocols we describe are intended as educational reference points, not clinical prescriptions. In clinical practice, they must be implemented by a qualified, experienced practitioner who is continuously monitoring and adapting.

References — Chapter Six

Greenberg, L.M. & Waldman, I.D. (1993). 'Developmental normative data on the Test of Variables of Attention (TOVA).' Journal of Child Psychology and Psychiatry, 34(6), 1019–1030.

Leark, R.A. et al. (1996). 'TOVA professional manual.' Los Alamitos, CA: Universal Attention Disorders.

Tinius, T.P. (2003). 'The Intermediate Visual and Auditory Continuous Performance Test as a neuropsychological measure.' Archives of Clinical Neuropsychology, 18(2), 199–214.

Amen, D.G. (2013). Healing ADD: The Breakthrough Program That Allows You to See and Heal the 7 Types of ADD (revised ed.). New York: Berkley Books.

Johnstone, J., Gunkelman, J. & Lunt, J. (2005). 'Clinical database development: characterization of EEG phenotypes.' Clinical EEG and Neuroscience, 36(2), 99–107.

Arns, M. et al. (2013). 'Evaluation of neurofeedback in ADHD: the long and winding road.' Biological Psychology, 95, 108–115.

Tye, C., McLoughlin, G., Kuntsi, J. & Asherson, P. (2011). 'Electrophysiological markers of genetic risk for ADHD.' Expert Reviews in Molecular Medicine, 13, e9.

Barkley, R.A. (2015). Attention-Deficit Hyperactivity Disorder: A Handbook for Diagnosis and Treatment (4th ed.). New York: Guilford Press.

Conners, C.K. (2008). Conners 3rd Edition. Toronto: Multi-Health Systems.

Wechsler, D. (2008). Wechsler Adult Intelligence Scale, Fourth Edition (WAIS-IV). San Antonio: Pearson.

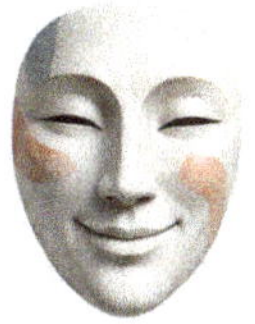

Chapter Seven

Type 1 — Classic ADHD

Too little activation, too much commotion

> ***LIAM — Age 25:*** *He is sitting in a waiting room that is not simply a doctor's office, for the first time in his life, about to have a brain assessment that is not a rating scale. He has been told it will take about forty minutes, involve a cap on his head, and be entirely painless. He is deeply sceptical. He is also, for reasons he cannot name, quietly hoping it tells him something. He is tired of explanations that explain nothing. He would like, just once, to see the actual problem.*

Classic ADHD — what Amen's typology calls Type 1, and what the DSM calls the Predominantly Hyperactive-Impulsive or Combined presentation — is the version of ADHD that most people picture when they hear the diagnosis. The bouncing child. The interrupted conversation. The unfinished project. The car parked half in the bay. It is the presentation that gets noticed, assessed, and treated earliest, because it is the presentation that makes everyone around the person uncomfortable.

It is also, neurologically speaking, the most straightforward of the seven subtypes — which does not mean it is simple, but does mean it is the presentation for which the research evidence is most extensive, the neurophysiological profile most consistently identified, and the treatment literature most developed. Understanding Classic ADHD well is the foundation for understanding what goes differently in each of the six types that follow.

The Symptom Cluster

Classic ADHD presents with the full combined symptom picture: prominent hyperactivity and impulsivity alongside significant inattention. The hyperactivity is not merely restlessness — it is a pervasive physical urgency, as though the body is constantly responding to an internal signal to move that has no external trigger. Liam, at nine, was sent out of class repeatedly for leaving his seat. At twenty-five, he manifests this as constant physical restlessness, an inability to remain seated for extended periods, habitual fidgeting, and a compulsive need to be doing something with his hands. The motor drive has not disappeared; it has adapted to an adult body in adult environments with marginally more social inhibition.

Impulsivity in Classic ADHD is similarly persistent: speaking before thinking, making decisions without adequate deliberation, difficulty waiting in queues or for a turn in conversation, and a characteristic pattern of action preceding consideration. The prefrontal brakes are genuinely delayed — not absent, but slow enough that the impulse arrives at expression before the evaluative process has completed. For Liam, this has produced a pattern of confrontations, lost jobs, and legal consequences that track the original impulse across twenty-five years of adult contexts.

The inattentive component coexists with the hyperactivity: difficulty sustaining attention on tasks that lack immediate novelty or urgency, frequent errors of omission (starting tasks and failing to complete them), difficulty tracking multi-step instructions, and a characteristic pattern of high performance under pressure — when the crisis provides sufficient arousal — and poor performance in the absence of that urgency. The Salience Network calibration described in Chapter Four is consistently visible in clinical presentation.

SPECT and QEEG Findings

SPECT imaging in Classic ADHD consistently shows decreased activity in the prefrontal cortex and the basal ganglia — particularly in the striatum — both at rest and during cognitive challenge. The prefrontal hypoperfusion reflects the underactivation of the central executive network that produces the characteristic difficulties with planning, inhibition, and sustained cognitive effort. When asked to concentrate, the prefrontal cortex of Classic ADHD actually activates less rather than more — the paradox that explains why effort alone cannot substitute for the neurological drive to focus (Amen, 2013).

QEEG in Classic ADHD shows the most reliably replicated pattern in the ADHD literature: elevated theta power (4–8 Hz) in frontal and central regions, reduced beta power (13–30 Hz) across the cortex, and a characteristic elevation of the theta/beta ratio (TBR) that reflects cortical underactivation. The theta excess is particularly pronounced at Fz (frontal midline) and Cz (central midline) sites in the international 10-20 electrode placement system. In the combined presentation, elevated theta may extend into parietal regions, reflecting the broader network underactivation.

Alpha peak frequency in Classic ADHD is often at the low end of the normal range or slightly below, reflecting the overall slowing of cortical processing speed. Event-related potentials — particularly the P300 amplitude, which indexes the allocation of attentional resources to target stimuli — are reliably reduced, and P300 latency (reflecting processing speed) is reliably prolonged (Tye et al., 2011).

Importantly, stimulant medication in individuals with the Classic ADHD QEEG profile produces measurable normalisation of these patterns: theta power reduces, beta power increases, TBR decreases toward the normal range, and P300 amplitude and latency normalise. This provides objective biological confirmation that the medication is having its intended neurophysiological effect — and equally, when repeated QEEG over time shows attenuation of these medication effects, it provides early objective evidence of pharmacodynamic tolerance.

Classic ADHD
(excess frontal theta)

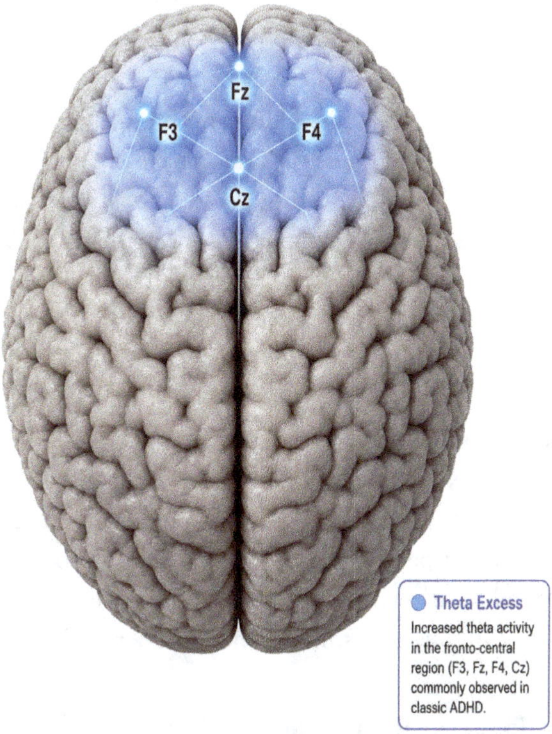

Neurochemical Profile and Genetic Correlates

Classic ADHD is the presentation most closely associated with the mesocortical dopaminergic hypothesis: reduced dopaminergic tone in the pathway from the ventral tegmental area to the prefrontal cortex, resulting in insufficient activation of the reward-prediction machinery that drives sustained effortful attention. The DAT1 gene — encoding the dopamine transporter — is among the most replicated molecular genetic findings in ADHD, with specific variants associated with slower clearance of dopamine from the synapse and consequently altered dopaminergic signalling (Faraone & Larsson, 2019).

DRD4 variants — particularly the 7-repeat allele of the DRD4 exon III VNTR — have been associated with Classic ADHD and specifically with novelty-seeking and impulsivity, consistent with the clinical profile. These variants appear to reduce the sensitivity of the D4 receptor, requiring greater dopaminergic stimulation to produce equivalent signalling — which maps elegantly onto the clinical observation that Classic ADHD brains require higher levels of novelty, stimulation, or urgency to achieve adequate prefrontal activation.

Noradrenergic contributions are also well-documented in this profile: the NET1 gene, encoding the noradrenaline transporter, has been associated with ADHD in several studies, and the noradrenergic pathway's role in signal-to-noise optimisation in prefrontal circuits is directly relevant to the Classic ADHD pattern of responding well to stimulation and poorly to monotony.

What Classic ADHD Is Confused With — and How to Distinguish

The most common diagnostic confusion in Classic ADHD involves three conditions that share significant symptom overlap with the combined presentation.

Bipolar disorder — particularly the hypomanic presentation — can look remarkably similar to Classic ADHD in cross-sectional assessment: elevated energy, decreased need for sleep, rapid speech, impulsivity, distractibility, and inflated self-esteem. The critical distinctions are temporal: bipolar disorder involves episodic fluctuations in state, typically lasting days to weeks, with clear periods of return to baseline mood and energy between episodes.

ADHD symptoms are persistent, present from childhood, and relatively constant in severity (though with considerable situational variation). QEEG helps here: the cortical underactivation pattern of Classic ADHD is distinct from the elevated high-beta that may accompany hypomanic states. A careful developmental history is essential.

Anxiety disorders produce attentional difficulties, restlessness, and impaired concentration that can resemble hyperactive ADHD. The distinction — again, critical for treatment — lies in the direction of neurophysiological arousal: anxiety involves overactivation of threat-detection circuitry, typically visible as elevated high-beta on QEEG, while Classic ADHD involves underactivation of the frontal executive system visible as elevated theta. Both produce distractibility; the mechanisms are opposite. In children, hyperactive behaviour driven by anxiety typically shows greater situational specificity (worse in novel or evaluative situations) than ADHD-driven hyperactivity (which is more pervasive across contexts).

Substance use, particularly stimulant use, can produce hyperactive and impulsive behaviour that mimics ADHD. Careful history about substance use patterns and the timeline relative to symptom onset is essential. Importantly, the CPT/QEEG assessment should be conducted after an appropriate washout period from any active substances.

Medication Implications

Classic ADHD has the strongest evidence base for stimulant medication response of any ADHD subtype. The elevated TBR/frontal theta profile is the QEEG pattern most predictive of a positive methylphenidate or amphetamine response (Arns et al., 2013). Both long-acting methylphenidate (Concerta, Ritalin LA) and mixed amphetamine salts (Adderall XR) or lisdexamfetamine (Vyvanse) are evidence-based options, with individual response and side-effect profiles guiding selection.

The key clinical caution, established in Chapter Five, is that stimulant benefit in Classic ADHD is primarily short-to-medium term. The pharmacological tolerance that develops with sustained use is most clearly documented in the Classic presentation — the profile for which stimulant response is initially strongest, but for which the DAT upregulation that underlies tolerance is also most pronounced. Objective monitoring with periodic CPT or QEEG re-assessment provides the most reliable means of detecting tolerance before it produces clinical deterioration.

Non-stimulant medications — atomoxetine (Strattera), guanfacine (Intuniv), bupropion — are second-line options with a different mechanism and typically lower efficacy in the Classic presentation than stimulants, but important for individuals who cannot tolerate stimulants or for whom controlled-substance prescribing is contraindicated.

Supplement Targets

Several nutritional factors have documented relevance to the dopaminergic and noradrenergic systems implicated in Classic ADHD.

Iron (specifically serum ferritin) is among the best-documented nutritional correlates of ADHD severity: multiple studies have found that children with ADHD have significantly lower ferritin levels than typically developing controls, and that iron supplementation in iron-deficient children produces measurable improvements in attentional performance and ADHD rating scores. Ferritin levels below 30 ng/mL — a threshold often within the 'normal' reference range — are associated with increased ADHD symptom severity and poorer cognitive performance. Functional testing of ferritin level should be part of any integrative ADHD assessment (Konofal et al., 2004; Greenblatt, 2017).

Zinc is a cofactor in dopamine synthesis and metabolism, and reduced zinc levels have been found in multiple studies of children with ADHD. Zinc supplementation, particularly in conjunction with stimulant medication, has been shown in some trials to reduce the dose of stimulant required for symptom control. Magnesium deficiency, common in ADHD populations, affects both dopaminergic and noradrenergic signalling and is associated with hyperactivity and sleep disturbance. Magnesium glycinate supplementation is well-tolerated and has a small but documented evidence base for symptom reduction.

Omega-3 fatty acids, particularly EPA and DHA, are required for normal dopamine receptor function and membrane fluidity in neural tissue. Meta-analyses have found a modest but significant effect of omega-3 supplementation on ADHD symptoms, with effect sizes smaller than those of medication but clinically meaningful as an adjunct (Bloch & Mulqueen, 2014). The combination of EPA-rich omega-3 with adequate zinc and iron forms a rational nutritional foundation for Classic ADHD management.

Neurofeedback Protocol Overview

The neurofeedback protocol historically most associated with Classic ADHD is theta suppression combined with beta enhancement at frontal and central sites (typically Fz and Cz) — training the brain to reduce its excess slow-wave activity and increase the faster, more engaged processing associated with sustained attention. This protocol emerged from the foundational research of Lubar and colleagues in the 1970s and has been refined through decades of clinical application.

However, as noted in Chapter Six, protocols must be adapted continuously as the brain changes. Modern QEEG-guided approaches may also incorporate training at additional sites, coherence training to normalise inter-regional connectivity, and alpha peak frequency training in individuals whose slow alpha peak contributes to the overall pattern of cortical slowing. The detailed protocol design requires ongoing QEEG monitoring by a BCIA-accredited neurofeedback practitioner with QEEG competency — the overview here is intended to convey the neurophysiological logic, not to serve as a clinical protocol.

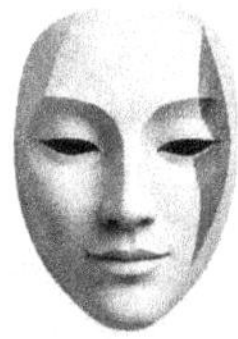

Chapter Eight
Type 2 — Inattentive ADHD

The brain that has slipped away before you noticed it was gone

> ***PRIYA — Age 27:*** *She has been asked to complete a TOVA as part of her assessment. She sits at the computer for twenty-two minutes, and the results are unambiguous: significant elevation in omission errors (missed targets), elevated response time variability (inconsistent attention), and a pattern most pronounced in the first, low-frequency half of the test — when target frequency is low and sustained vigilance is most demanding. Her commission errors are not significantly elevated. She is not impulsive. She is absent. The test has, for the first time in twenty-seven years, measured the actual problem.*

Inattentive ADHD — Type 2 in Amen's framework, and the Predominantly Inattentive presentation in DSM-5 — is the invisible version. No disruption. No chair-climbing. No blurted answers. Just a mind that has drifted to somewhere quieter and more interesting than the task at hand, in ways that nobody notices until the consequences accumulate.

It is, paradoxically, often the most debilitating form in adult life. The Classic ADHD child who disrupts the classroom will, at minimum, receive attention — clinical attention, parental attention, school intervention, sometimes punitive attention, but attention nonetheless. The Inattentive child drifts through education essentially undetected, accumulating a growing gap between their intellectual potential and their actual achievement, while their teachers write 'could try harder' and their parents assume they are simply dreamers. By the time the consequences become undeniable, years of unnecessary difficulty have already elapsed.

The Symptom Cluster

Inattentive ADHD presents primarily through failures of sustained attention rather than through hyperactivity or impulsivity. The characteristic experience is of a mind that will not stay where it is directed: wandering off task without warning, returning without the person having experienced the departure, producing the maddening situation in which effort and result are chronically decoupled.

Key features include persistent difficulty sustaining attention on tasks that are not immediately engaging; frequent mind-wandering that the individual often does not notice until sometime after it has occurred; difficulty following multi-step verbal instructions, because attention is lost partway through the sequence; consistent failure to complete tasks despite having begun them; a tendency to be detail-blind — missing important elements of tasks, instructions, or communications that were present but did not register; and a specific vulnerability in listening comprehension, where spoken information is more likely to be lost than written information.

Absent from this picture, characteristically, is significant hyperactivity. The Inattentive individual is typically quiet, often described as 'calm' or 'passive,' sometimes perceived as shy or slow when they are neither. Physical restlessness, if present, is subtle — a tendency to fidget with small objects, a preference for activity over stillness, but without the dramatic motor drive of Classic ADHD. The impulsivity of Classic ADHD is also typically absent or much less prominent, which is why the CPT profile shows elevated omissions (missed targets, reflecting inattention) without significantly elevated commissions (false alarms, reflecting impulsivity).

In adults, inattentive ADHD commonly presents with a history of underachievement despite adequate intelligence; a pattern of losing things, missing appointments, and forgetting obligations; difficulty with self-initiated tasks in the absence of external structure; and frequently a sense of internal chaos behind an apparently organised exterior — particularly in women who have developed sophisticated compensatory strategies at significant cognitive cost.

SPECT and QEEG Findings

SPECT imaging in Inattentive ADHD shows a pattern that overlaps with Classic ADHD — prefrontal hypoperfusion — but with several distinguishing features. The underactivation in the inattentive profile tends to be more pronounced in the parietal regions, reflecting impairment of the sustained attention networks that include the right parietal cortex and posterior attention system. During cognitive challenge, activation may actually decrease further rather than increasing — the 'paradoxical deactivation' that characterises ADHD-related prefrontal underactivation.

QEEG in Inattentive ADHD characteristically shows elevated frontal alpha rather than elevated frontal theta — a critically important distinction. Alpha frequencies (8–12 Hz) represent the brain's idling rhythm: the pattern of coordinated oscillation that predominates when the brain is disengaged from active cognitive processing. In neurotypical individuals, alpha is suppressed during tasks requiring focused attention — a phenomenon called alpha desynchronisation. In the Inattentive ADHD profile, alpha suppression is impaired: the brain maintains its idling rhythm even when active engagement is demanded, producing the neurological equivalent of a car that remains in neutral regardless of how much fuel is applied.

This distinction — theta excess in Classic ADHD versus alpha excess in Inattentive ADHD — has profound treatment implications. The frontal theta excess profile responds well to stimulant medication, which increases cortical arousal and normalises the TBR. The frontal alpha excess profile — Priya's pattern — responds less consistently to stimulants, and in some cases stimulants increase alpha rather than reducing it, worsening the very pattern they are intended to address. The alpha-excess profile responds more specifically to neurofeedback protocols targeting frontal alpha suppression.

A particularly important variant within the Inattentive type involves slowing of the alpha peak frequency (APF) — the dominant frequency within the alpha band. Normal APF for adults is approximately 10 Hz. Slowing to 8–9 Hz or below is associated with reduced processing speed, greater task-engagement difficulty, and stronger treatment resistance to both stimulants and standard theta-suppression neurofeedback protocols. This variant — which Johnstone and Gunkelman identified as a distinct EEG phenotype requiring specific protocol modification — may explain a significant proportion of inattentive ADHD cases that fail to respond to standard interventions.

Inattentive ADHD
(excess frontal alpha)

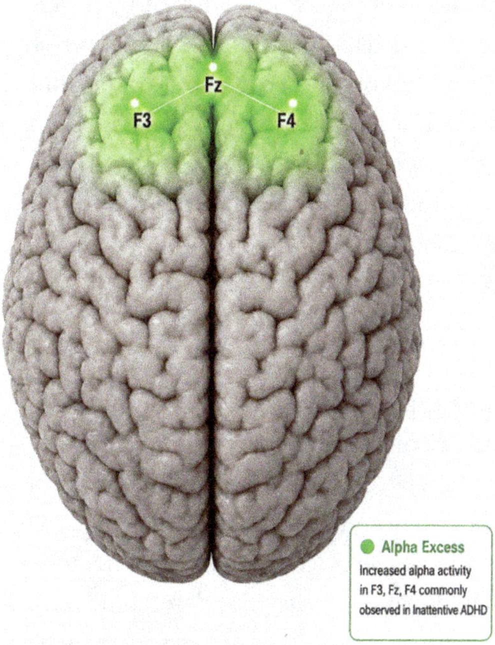

Neurochemical Profile and the Gender Dimension

The Inattentive presentation has somewhat different neurochemical associations than the Classic type. Dopaminergic involvement is present but may be less central than in Classic ADHD: the parietal underactivation pattern is more closely associated with cholinergic dysfunction, and the alpha-excess profile is associated with serotoninergic as well as dopaminergic modulation. Some research has found lower serotonin metabolite levels in inattentive ADHD populations compared to combined type (Halmøy et al., 2010).

Iron deficiency — measured as low serum ferritin — is consistently associated with greater overall ADHD symptom severity, with low ferritin found in up to 84% of children with ADHD compared to 18% of controls; ferritin levels correlate inversely with symptom severity regardless of subtype (Konofal et al., 2004). Ferritin testing is therefore clinically relevant across all ADHD presentations, not specifically the Inattentive type. Vitamin D deficiency, however, has been more specifically associated with attentional difficulties, and supplementation in deficient individuals has shown modest but significant benefits for attention (Mohammadpour et al., 2018).

The gender dimension of inattentive ADHD deserves particular emphasis. Women are overrepresented in the inattentive presentation relative to men, and are consequently overrepresented in the population that reaches adulthood without a correct diagnosis. The oestrogen-dopamine interaction — oestrogen modulates dopamine release and receptor sensitivity — means that inattentive ADHD symptoms in women fluctuate with hormonal cycles in ways that have only recently begun to receive systematic clinical attention. Symptoms commonly worsen in the luteal phase of the menstrual cycle, during perimenopause, and following childbirth — periods of reduced oestrogen availability that transiently reduce dopaminergic tone. This pattern, when recognised, has direct implications for both assessment timing and treatment approach.

What Inattentive ADHD Is Confused With

The quiet, non-disruptive presentation of Inattentive ADHD creates distinctive confusion patterns. The three most clinically important are depression, anxiety, and giftedness.

Depression and inattentive ADHD are frequently confused and frequently co-occur. Both produce difficulty concentrating, psychomotor slowing, reduced motivation, and poor task completion. The critical distinctions are developmental (ADHD symptoms present from childhood; depressive episodes have a characteristic onset) and neurophysiological (depression typically shows frontal alpha asymmetry with greater relative left-frontal alpha, while inattentive ADHD shows a more diffuse frontal alpha excess). The therapeutic implications differ substantially: antidepressants alone will not address ADHD, and ADHD alone — particularly the inattentive presentation — can look clinically indistinguishable from mild-moderate depression.

Anxiety, as noted in Chapter Three, produces similar attentional difficulties through a completely different mechanism. The anxious brain's difficulty concentrating arises from competition between task-directed attention and threat-monitoring processes — not from cortical underactivation. QEEG again provides the clearest distinction: anxiety shows elevated high-beta; inattentive ADHD shows elevated alpha.

Perhaps the most underappreciated confusion is with giftedness. Intellectually gifted individuals in educational environments that do not challenge them can look remarkably like inattentive ADHD: bored, inattentive, producing work well below their capability, and described by teachers as 'not working to potential.' The critical clinical question is whether the attentional difficulties are pervasive across all contexts (suggesting ADHD) or specific to unchallenging environments (suggesting inadequate educational placement). CPT performance in gifted-but-unstimulated children is often entirely normal — another argument for objective neurophysiological assessment alongside the behavioural measures.

Medication and Supplement Implications

As noted above, stimulant response in Inattentive ADHD is less consistently positive than in Classic ADHD. Some individuals respond well; others show minimal benefit or adverse effects. The alpha-excess QEEG profile is less reliably predictive of stimulant response than the theta-excess profile, and the presence of slowed APF is associated with particularly poor stimulant response. Non-stimulants, including atomoxetine, may be preferable for some individuals with this profile.

Nutritional priorities include iron (ferritin testing is essential), vitamin D (supplementation to achieve the 50–80 ng/mL range associated with optimal cognitive function), omega-3 fatty acids, and zinc. N-acetylcysteine (NAC), which supports glutamate regulation and has antioxidant properties, has emerging evidence for inattentive symptoms and may be particularly relevant in the alpha-excess profile. Magnesium glycinate addresses the sleep difficulties that frequently accompany and worsen the inattentive presentation.

Neurofeedback Protocol Overview

Neurofeedback for the Inattentive type targets frontal alpha suppression — training the brain to desynchronise its alpha rhythm during cognitive engagement — rather than the theta suppression that is appropriate for Classic ADHD. For individuals with slowed APF, the approach additionally incorporates protocols targeting alpha peak frequency upshift, which Gunkelman's phenotype framework identifies as requiring specific training parameters distinct from standard alpha-suppression work.

The alpha-suppression protocol requires a clinician who can distinguish alpha excess from theta excess on the QEEG, identify the peak frequency accurately, and differentiate the Inattentive profile from the Slowed APF variant — distinctions that require QEEG expertise and cannot be made from CPT results or clinical presentation alone. This is an example of why BCIA accreditation with QEEG competency is not merely a professional credential but a clinical necessity for safe and effective neurofeedback delivery.

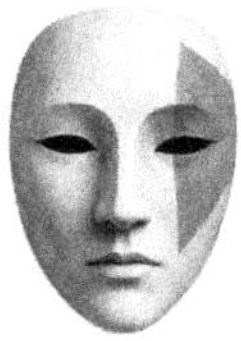

Chapter Nine

Type 3 — Overfocused ADHD

When the brake won't release — and focus becomes a prison

> ***OLIVER — Age 34:*** *He is explaining to the couples therapist, patiently and in considerable detail, why he is correct about the kitchen renovation. He has been explaining this for thirty-seven minutes. The therapist has attempted to redirect the conversation four times. Oliver is aware of all four attempts. He has filed them away and continued. He does not experience this as a problem. He experiences it as thoroughness. His wife, across the room, is looking at the wall.*

Overfocused ADHD is the type that most confuses people — including clinicians — precisely because its central feature appears, at first glance, to be the opposite of attention deficit. These are individuals who can focus intensely, sometimes for hours without interruption. They complete tasks to a degree of thoroughness that would exhaust most people. They notice details that others miss. They hold positions with a tenacity that their colleagues find either admirable or maddening, depending on the day.

What they cannot do is shift. They are not attention-deficient. They are attention-rigid: locked onto a thought, a task, an opinion, or a concern in ways that no amount of social feedback, rational argument, or practical necessity can easily dislodge. The problem is not that attention won't start. It is that it won't stop.

The Symptom Cluster

Overfocused ADHD is characterised by cognitive inflexibility rather than inattention, and by intensity of focus rather than brevity of it. The hallmark symptoms include: excessive or compulsive worry that is difficult to interrupt; cognitive rigidity — difficulty changing plans, accommodating new information, or accepting that a different approach might be equally valid; an intense need for order and routine, with significant distress when routines are disrupted; oppositional, argumentative behaviour that feels to the individual like principled consistency rather than inflexibility; compulsive re-reading, re-checking, or re-doing of work that is already sufficient; difficulty transitioning between tasks, even when the transition is clearly appropriate; and a tendency to hold grudges disproportionately, because the cognitive loop that would normally allow emotional resolution keeps restarting.

This cluster frequently leads to misdiagnosis as obsessive-compulsive disorder — and the two conditions can co-occur. The critical clinical distinction is that OCD involves ego-dystonic intrusions (the compulsions feel foreign and unwanted to the person) while Overfocused ADHD involves ego-syntonic perseveration (the person's tenacity feels appropriate and even virtuous to them). Oliver does not experience his thirty-seven-minute kitchen renovation monologue as a problem. He experiences it as necessary. This is, neurologically speaking, an important distinction.

In children, Overfocused ADHD often presents as oppositional behaviour, difficulty transitioning between activities, compulsive arguing, and strong resistance to direction — not because the child is defiant in the wilful sense, but because the anterior cingulate cortex that should process task switching and allow errors to be corrected and plans to be updated is firing in ways that make letting go neurologically difficult.

SPECT and QEEG Findings

The distinctive feature of Overfocused ADHD on SPECT is not, as in Classic ADHD, a hypoperfused prefrontal cortex, but a hyperperfused anterior cingulate cortex (ACC). The ACC — sitting at the junction between the prefrontal cortex and the limbic system — plays a critical role in error detection, conflict monitoring, and cognitive flexibility: it is the system that registers when a behaviour is producing unwanted outcomes and signals the need for an adjustment. In Overfocused ADHD, this system is overactive, generating a continuous sense of internal conflict, urgency, and incompleteness that drives the perseverative behaviour and the compulsive quality of the focus. The brake is not released because the ACC keeps signalling that the current task requires more attention.

QEEG in Overfocused ADHD shows a characteristic pattern of elevated high-beta activity (typically 20–30 Hz) in the frontal midline and anterior cingulate region, often accompanied by a relative reduction in alpha — the brain's deactivation signal — in the same areas. This is the neurophysiological pattern of a brain that is running too fast, too engaged, unable to shift down into the lower frequencies associated with mental flexibility and relaxation. Unlike Classic ADHD's slow theta excess, Overfocused ADHD shows fast-wave excess — a pattern that immediately distinguishes it from the Classic type and has entirely different treatment implications.

A further QEEG distinction worth noting involves the relationship between frontal alpha and obsessive behaviours. Some studies have found elevated resting frontotemporal alpha in individuals with OCD-spectrum presentations, with higher alpha power — reflecting cortical hypoactivation — proposed as a vulnerability marker for obsessive tendencies (Bucci et al., 2004; Ischebeck et al., 2014). This superficially resembles the frontal alpha excess of Inattentive ADHD, and might appear to overlap with the Overfocused pattern. The distinction is clinically and mechanistically important. In Overfocused ADHD, the pathological signature is elevated high-beta at frontal midline and anterior cingulate sites — a pattern of cortical overactivation and excessive engagement, reflecting a circuit that is running too hot and too fast to release its grip on the current cognitive object. The frontal alpha associated with OCD vulnerability reflects the opposite state: cortical underactivation, insufficient inhibitory control over intrusive thoughts, and a prefrontal cortex that is not adequately engaged to suppress unwanted mental content. In plain terms, Overfocused ADHD involves a brain that is locked on because it is too activated to let go. OCD-spectrum frontal hypoactivity involves a brain that cannot suppress intrusions because it is insufficiently activated to do so. The behaviours converge — perseveration, difficulty shifting — but the mechanisms are opposite, and the neurofeedback implications are opposite accordingly: Overfocused ADHD requires downtraining of excess fast waves, while the frontal hypoactivity pattern may benefit from uptraining of cortical engagement. Applying the wrong protocol to either pattern would be counterproductive.

Some individuals with Overfocused ADHD also show elevated coherence — excessive synchronisation of electrical activity between brain regions — in frontal circuits, suggesting that the perseverative behaviour has a network basis: circuits that should fire independently are locked together, preventing the flexible switching between mental sets that flexible cognition requires.

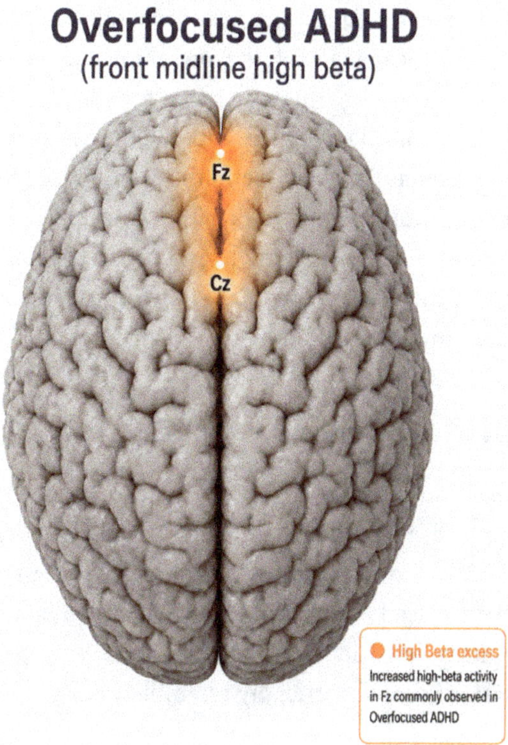

Neurochemical Profile

Overfocused ADHD is the subtype most clearly associated with serotonergic rather than primarily dopaminergic dysregulation. The ACC is rich in serotonin receptors, and serotonin plays a critical role in behavioural flexibility, the regulation of repetitive behaviour, and the inhibition of perseverative responses. The excess ACC activity in Overfocused ADHD is consistent with a profile of insufficient serotonergic inhibition of the cognitive loops that drive perseveration.

This has direct and important treatment implications: stimulants, which primarily increase dopaminergic tone, may worsen Overfocused ADHD by increasing the intensity of the already overactive ACC circuits. Clinical experience, and the neurophysiological logic of the presentation, both suggest that serotonin-supporting interventions are more appropriate as the primary pharmacological approach. SSRIs, which increase serotonin availability, are sometimes helpful. More targeted serotonergic supplements — 5-HTP (the immediate precursor to serotonin), inositol (which modulates serotonin receptor sensitivity), and L-tryptophan — have evidence bases in OCD and related presentations that are relevant here.

What Overfocused ADHD Is Confused With

Obsessive-compulsive disorder is the primary diagnostic confusion, as noted above. The ego-syntonic/ego-dystonic distinction is clinically useful but not always clean — individuals with Overfocused ADHD may develop secondary distress about their rigidity once its consequences become apparent, creating presentations that superficially resemble OCD.

A related but distinct diagnostic consideration is anankastic personality disorder (also called obsessive-compulsive personality disorder, OCPD) — a condition characterised by pervasive preoccupation with orderliness, perfectionism, and control that is longstanding, ego-syntonic, and present across virtually all domains of functioning. The surface overlap with Overfocused ADHD is considerable: both involve rigidity, difficulty delegating, excessive devotion to productivity, and strong resistance to changing established routines. The distinctions, however, are neurobiologically and clinically meaningful. Anankastic personality disorder involves a characterological pattern of control that is motivated by anxiety about disorder and imperfection

— the person holds on tightly because letting go feels dangerous. Overfocused ADHD involves a neurologically driven inability to shift cognitive set — the person cannot let go because the anterior cingulate cortex keeps signalling that the current task or thought is unfinished, regardless of any conscious desire to move on. The motivation is fundamentally different even when the behaviour looks the same. A further distinguishing feature is the attentional profile: individuals with anankastic personality disorder typically do not show the broader attentional difficulties, time blindness, or working memory impairments that characterise ADHD, and their hyperfocus on detail serves their perfectionist goals rather than occurring as an involuntary absorption independent of goal-relevance. On QEEG, anankastic personality disorder does not reliably produce the anterior cingulate high-beta excess that characterises Overfocused ADHD — a distinction that is invisible on any rating scale or clinical interview, but clear on neurophysiological assessment.

Autism spectrum disorder also overlaps substantially with Overfocused ADHD in presentation: restricted interests, cognitive inflexibility, strong preference for routine, difficulty with transitions, and social difficulties secondary to communication rigidity. QEEG can contribute to the distinction — ASD shows coherence abnormalities in characteristic patterns that differ from those of Overfocused ADHD — but clinical judgment and developmental history remain essential.

Perfectionism and workaholism, particularly in high-achieving adults, can mask Overfocused ADHD entirely. Oliver's colleagues know him as meticulous and brilliant. They do not know that his meticulousness costs him three times as long as equivalent work costs his peers, and that the cost is not additional quality but additional compulsion.

Medication and Supplement Implications

As emphasised above, stimulant medications are not the appropriate first-line approach for Overfocused ADHD and may significantly worsen the presentation by increasing the intensity of already overactive anterior cingulate circuits. When stimulants are clinically indicated for co-occurring attentional difficulties, they should be introduced cautiously, at low doses, with careful monitoring for worsening of rigidity, worry, or compulsive behaviour.

Serotonin-supporting approaches are the primary targets. 5-HTP supplementation (50–100 mg, typically taken in the evening) supports serotonin synthesis and may reduce the perseverative quality of the presentation. Inositol, at doses of 12–18 g per day, has demonstrated efficacy in OCD in controlled trials and is relevant to the Overfocused profile. Magnesium — which modulates glutamate activity and NMDA receptor function in the ACC — may help reduce the hyperactivity of the ACC circuits. Exercise, particularly aerobic exercise, is one of the most powerful serotonin-modulating interventions available and has a strong evidence base for its effects on cognitive flexibility.

Neurofeedback Protocol Overview

Neurofeedback for Overfocused ADHD targets reduction of the elevated high-beta excess in frontal midline and anterior cingulate sites, combined with alpha enhancement in these regions to support the shift toward mental flexibility. This is sometimes described as 'downtraining' the fast waves associated with excessive cognitive engagement, while training the alpha rhythms associated with a more relaxed, flexible cognitive state.

This protocol is the opposite, in important respects, of the protocol appropriate for Classic ADHD — another illustration of why QEEG-guided protocol design is essential, and why applying the same neurofeedback protocol to all ADHD presentations would be both ineffective and potentially harmful.

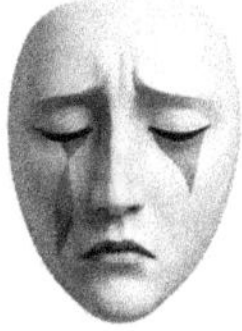

Chapter Ten

Type 4 — Temporal Lobe ADHD

The brain that can't read the room — or keep its own history straight

> ***DANIEL — Age 42:*** *He is describing, to the QEEG practitioner, the experience of sitting in meetings and being unable to follow the sequence of what is being said — not because he is distracted in the usual sense, but because the thread of the conversation seems to lose coherence partway through, as though sentences that should connect don't quite join. He has assumed for thirty years that this was a concentration problem. The practitioner is looking at his QEEG, noting the asymmetric temporal abnormalities, and suggesting it might be something more specific than that.*

The temporal lobes — sitting above the ears on both sides of the brain — are not a region that most people associate with ADHD. They are more commonly associated with memory (hippocampus), language (left temporal cortex), and emotion recognition (right temporal cortex). Which is precisely why Temporal Lobe ADHD is so frequently misdiagnosed, so persistently confusing, and so consequential when it goes unrecognised.

In Temporal Lobe ADHD, the attentional difficulties that produce the ADHD presentation arise not from frontal underactivation but from temporal instability — abnormal electrical activity in regions responsible for memory consolidation, auditory processing, and emotional interpretation. The result is a presentation that looks like ADHD on a rating scale but has a fundamentally different neurological basis — and a very different appropriate treatment.

The Symptom Cluster

Temporal Lobe ADHD presents with a distinctive cluster that combines attentional symptoms with features more characteristic of temporal dysfunction: difficulty with sequential processing (following multi-step verbal instructions, tracking conversations, reading sequences of events accurately); memory difficulties that go beyond the working memory deficits of Classic ADHD, extending into episodic memory (difficulty forming or retrieving autobiographical memories); a tendency to misread social situations or emotional cues, producing interpersonal difficulties; irritability and mood lability that is relatively rapid-cycling — not the sustained mood episodes of bipolar disorder, but the shorter-duration irritability associated with temporal instability; déjà vu experiences and occasionally brief dissociative episodes; and word-finding difficulties, particularly under stress.

Daniel's primary presentation — the inability to follow conversational sequences, the serial pattern of leaving jobs before they can end badly, the midnight rumination on decades-old conversations — reflects a temporal profile in which auditory sequential processing is impaired and emotional memories are processed with distorted intensity. He does not have poor memory for events; he has a temporal lobe that stores and retrieves emotional memories in ways that give old hurts disproportionate current vividness while allowing the pragmatic details of the present — the deadline, the meeting topic, the colleague's instruction — to fail to consolidate.

SPECT and QEEG Findings

SPECT in Temporal Lobe ADHD shows focal abnormalities in one or both temporal lobes — areas of decreased perfusion, asymmetric activation, or in some cases scattered areas of increased activity associated with temporal lobe micro-seizure activity. Right temporal abnormalities are associated with social difficulties and emotional processing impairment; left temporal abnormalities with language processing, word-finding, and auditory sequential processing difficulties. The presence of temporal abnormalities distinguishes this profile from the frontal patterns of Classic or Inattentive ADHD.

QEEG in Temporal Lobe ADHD shows temporal slow waves — excess theta or delta in temporal regions (T3, T4, T5, T6 in the 10-20 system) — which may be symmetric or asymmetric. In cases with more significant instability, there may be episodic temporal spiking or bursting — brief paroxysmal discharges that do not meet the threshold for clinical epilepsy but represent excess temporal excitability. This pattern is particularly important to identify because it has direct implications for medication selection: stimulants can lower seizure threshold and may worsen temporal instability in some individuals with this profile.

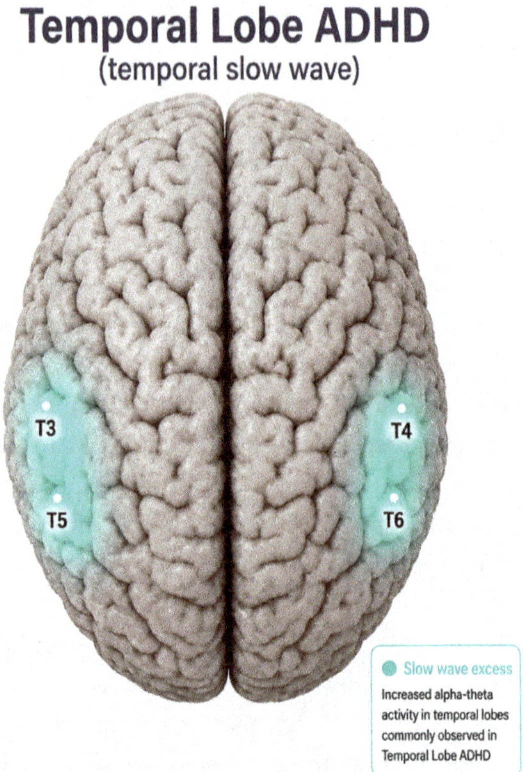

Neurochemical Profile and Differential Considerations

The neurochemical picture in Temporal Lobe ADHD is more complex than the primarily dopaminergic/noradrenergic profile of Classic ADHD. Gamma-aminobutyric acid (GABA) — the brain's primary inhibitory neurotransmitter — plays a critical role in temporal lobe stability, suppressing excess excitability and preventing the micro-discharge activity that characterises more extreme versions of this profile. GABA-supporting interventions are therefore particularly relevant here.

Temporal Lobe ADHD is the presentation most frequently confused with — and most frequently co-occurring with — mood disorders, specifically bipolar spectrum. The mood lability, the irritability, the rapid shifts between emotional states, and the tendency to misinterpret social cues all resemble bipolar spectrum presentations. The key distinction is that the mood changes in Temporal Lobe ADHD are typically shorter in duration (minutes to hours rather than days), more often triggered by specific stimuli, and more clearly linked to temporal instability rather than to the circadian and biological rhythms that drive bipolar cycling. QEEG and SPECT findings — temporal rather than whole-cortex pattern — help make the distinction.

Traumatic brain injury and post-concussive syndrome produce patterns that overlap substantially with Temporal Lobe ADHD on both QEEG and SPECT. A careful head injury history should be part of any assessment where the temporal profile is present. Chronic migraine — which has temporal lobe correlates — is also relevant to consider.

Medication and Supplement Implications

The medication approach to Temporal Lobe ADHD requires greater caution than the Classic type. Stimulants can be used but should be introduced cautiously; if temporal instability is significant on QEEG, temporal stabilisation should be the priority before introducing agents that may lower seizure threshold. Anticonvulsants — particularly valproate, lamotrigine, and gabapentin — are sometimes used in temporal lobe presentations, particularly where mood lability and episodic dyscontrol are prominent. On the other hand, levetiracetam can worsen mood instability.

GABA-supporting supplements are the nutritional priority: magnesium glycinate (which modulates GABA receptor function), L-theanine (which increases GABA activity and promotes alpha synchrony), and taurine (an inhibitory neuromodulator with GABA-like properties) are all relevant. Zinc and omega-3 fatty acids support the broader neurochemical environment. B6 (pyridoxine) is an important cofactor in GABA synthesis and has specific relevance in this profile.

Neurofeedback Protocol Overview

Neurofeedback for Temporal Lobe ADHD targets temporal stabilisation: reducing excess slow-wave activity in temporal regions, increasing SMR (sensorimotor rhythm, 12–15 Hz) at temporal sites, and where appropriate, addressing coherence abnormalities between temporal and frontal regions. In cases with significant temporal instability, careful monitoring during neurofeedback is essential — rapid changes in temporal activity can occasionally produce transient mood lability that requires protocol adjustment. This is another presentation where QEEG expertise and clinical judgment from a BCIA-accredited practitioner are not optional and might also require close collaboration with a neurologist if indicated.

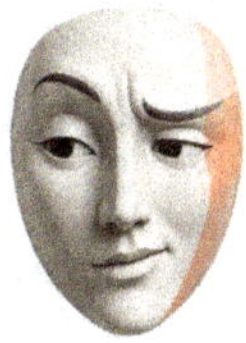

Chapter Eleven

Type 5 — Limbic ADHD

The brain that feels everything first and thinks about it later

> ***MAYA — Age 38:*** *She has just received her QEEG report. The clinician is explaining that her frontal alpha is elevated — particularly on the left side — and that her limbic system is showing heightened reactivity markers consistent with the pattern her emotional experience has always suggested. Maya reads the phrase 'elevated left frontal alpha with limbic hyperactivation' and, for the first time, stops feeling like a character flaw and starts feeling like a brain. 'Can it change?' she asks. The answer is yes.*

Limbic ADHD is the type that most clearly illustrates why the DSM's exclusion of emotional dysregulation from the ADHD criteria is not a minor diagnostic oversight. For individuals with this profile, the attentional difficulties are real and impairing — but they are substantially secondary to an emotional processing system that is chronically dysregulated, amplifying experiences of rejection, failure, loss, and uncertainty to a degree that overwhelms executive function and makes effective attention nearly impossible.

This is Maya's brain. It is the brain that processes every interaction through a system calibrated to respond to ordinary experiences with extraordinary intensity. The manager's neutral 'good work' that Maya hears as implicit 'not excellent enough.' The slight pause before a reply to a text message that reads, to Maya, as the beginning of a withdrawal. The emotional amplifier that has been set, since childhood, to a frequency the world around her does not recognise as rational — but which is, neurologically, entirely explicable.

The Symptom Cluster

Limbic ADHD presents with a primary picture of mood dysregulation combined with attentional difficulties. The core features include: chronic low-grade negative mood that is not the sustained sadness of major depression but a persistent emotional undertone of pessimism, heaviness, or low hedonic tone; heightened emotional reactivity — emotions arriving with greater intensity and less warning than the individual's context warrants; a strongly negative internal monologue, often described as a 'bully in the head'; difficulty recovering from negative emotional experiences, with rumination loops that sustain the emotional state well beyond its trigger; hypersensitivity to criticism, rejection, or perceived disappointment (the RSD dimension described in Chapter Two); and fatigue, not from physical exertion but from the sustained cognitive-emotional effort of managing a limbic system that is constantly overcontributing to every experience.

The attentional symptoms arise largely from the emotional overactivation: a limbic system in a state of chronic low-grade negative arousal competes with the prefrontal cortex for attentional resources, both directly (emotional preoccupation consumes working memory) and indirectly (negative mood reduces dopaminergic motivation and prefrontal engagement). The attention difficulties are real but secondary — which means that treatments targeting only the attentional symptoms will produce partial and temporary relief at best.

SPECT and QEEG Findings

SPECT in Limbic ADHD shows increased activity in the deep limbic system — the cingulate gyrus (particularly its anterior portion), the basal ganglia, and the amygdala — in conjunction with reduced activity in the prefrontal cortex. The limbic hyperactivation drives the chronic emotional preoccupation and negative mood; the prefrontal underactivation impairs the inhibitory regulation that would normally modulate limbic responses. The interaction between these two patterns produces the characteristic profile: emotional experience that is too intense, too persistent, and insufficiently regulated.

QEEG in Limbic ADHD characteristically shows elevated left frontal alpha— a pattern extensively studied in the context of depression and negative affect. The asymmetry is important: greater relative alpha power in the left frontal region (indicating lower left-frontal activation) compared to the right is associated with approach-withdrawal motivation imbalance, negative affective bias, and the chronic low-hedonic-tone that characterises this profile. This frontal alpha asymmetry pattern — which can be quantified as the alpha asymmetry index — distinguishes the Limbic type from other ADHD presentations and from standard depression, and provides a direct neurofeedback training target.

Limbic ADHD
(left frontal alpha)

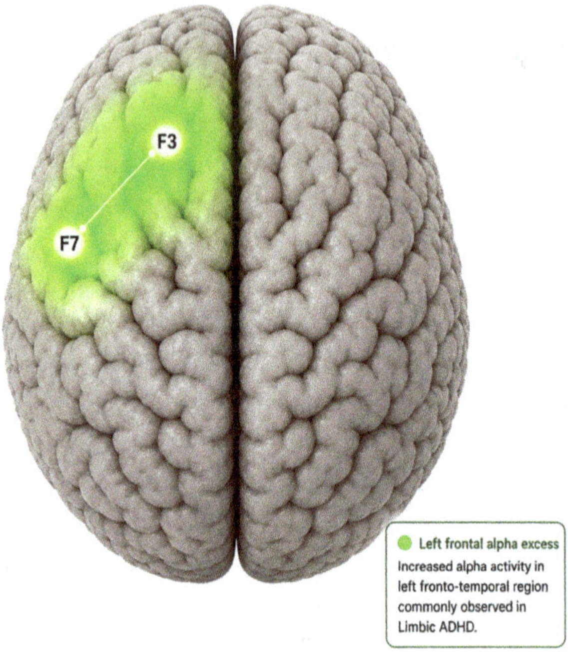

Neurochemical Profile

Limbic ADHD involves disturbances in both the dopaminergic and serotonergic systems, with limbic dopamine and serotonin both contributing to the mood and motivational dysregulation. The noradrenergic system's role in modulating arousal and emotional reactivity is also relevant. Glutamate excess in limbic circuits has been implicated in the hyperactivity of limbic processing — a target for GABA-supporting interventions.

Omega-3 fatty acids are among the most relevant supplements for this profile: EPA in particular has demonstrated antidepressant and mood-stabilising effects in controlled trials and is particularly relevant given the limbic hyperactivation and negative mood characteristics. S-adenosyl methionine (SAMe), which is involved in the methylation of monoamine neurotransmitters and has demonstrated antidepressant effects, is an evidence-based adjunct. L-tyrosine, a precursor to dopamine and noradrenaline, supports the dopaminergic motivation circuit that is characteristically underactive in this presentation. Zinc modulates both dopaminergic and serotonergic signalling and has demonstrated antidepressant properties in clinical studies.

What Limbic ADHD Is Confused With

Limbic ADHD is the most frequently misdiagnosed subtype of ADHD, primarily because its primary presenting features — low mood, emotional reactivity, hypersensitivity — are read as depression and treated accordingly. The clinical distinction is important: depression responds to antidepressant therapy targeting serotonergic and noradrenergic systems; Limbic ADHD requires treatment of both the limbic hyperactivation and the prefrontal underactivation, and antidepressants alone leave the attentional and dysregulatory dimensions unaddressed.

Borderline personality disorder shares emotional dysregulation, rejection sensitivity, and intense interpersonal responses with Limbic ADHD, and the two can co-occur. QEEG is helpful here: the specific frontal alpha asymmetry pattern of Limbic ADHD differs from the broader coherence abnormalities and impulse-control-related patterns seen in BPD. Developmental history — ADHD present from childhood versus BPD-related difficulties emerging in adolescence and early adulthood against a backdrop of attachment disruption — contributes to the distinction.

Medication and Supplement Implications

The medication landscape for Limbic ADHD is more complex than for the Classic type. Stimulants alone are insufficient and may worsen mood dysregulation in some individuals. The combination of a stimulant with an SSRI or SNRI — targeting both the attentional and the limbic-depressive dimensions — is a common approach, though it requires careful titration. Bupropion, which affects dopamine and noradrenaline but also has antidepressant properties, may be particularly well-suited to this profile as a single agent addressing multiple dimensions simultaneously.

Nutritional priorities include: EPA-rich omega-3s (at least 1–2 g EPA daily), zinc, SAMe in deficient individuals, and L-tyrosine as a dopaminergic support. Adequate B12 and folate are essential cofactors in the methylation of neurotransmitters. Assessment of methylation status through functional testing — including MTHFR variant testing — is relevant in this profile, as methylation deficiencies can significantly worsen the serotonergic and dopaminergic imbalances that drive the limbic pattern.

Neurofeedback Protocol Overview

Neurofeedback for Limbic ADHD targets the frontal alpha asymmetry: training to reduce relative left-frontal alpha and increase left-frontal activation. This protocol — sometimes called asymmetry training or affective neurofeedback — has a dedicated evidence base in depression research and is directly applicable to the Limbic ADHD profile. Training at Fp1 and Fp2 (prefrontal electrodes) to increase left-relative activation has shown antidepressant effects and may specifically address the approach-motivation deficit that underlies both the low hedonic tone and the attentional difficulties of this presentation.

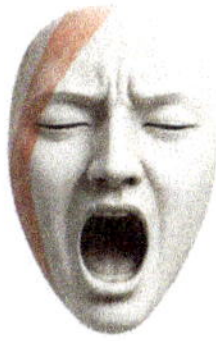

Chapter Twelve

Type 6 — Ring of Fire ADHD

The brain that can't turn down the volume on anything

> ***ZARA — Age 28:*** *She is sitting in the QEEG assessment room, and has asked whether the air conditioning can be turned down because the sound of the fan is interfering with her ability to think. The air conditioning is barely audible. The clinician turns it down. Zara's QEEG shows diffuse elevated high-beta across the entire cortex — the pattern the textbook calls Ring of Fire. 'What does this mean for medication?' she asks. The answer begins with 'not stimulants' and she starts crying, quietly, with relief.*

Ring of Fire ADHD is the presentation most likely to be harmed by the standard first-line treatment — and consequently the presentation most likely to arrive in a specialist's office in a state of iatrogenic deterioration, having been placed on stimulant after stimulant while becoming progressively more symptomatic.

It is named for the characteristic QEEG appearance: a ring of excess high-frequency activity encircling the cortex on a topographic map, typically visible from above as a roughly circular distribution of elevated beta power across frontal, temporal, parietal, and occipital regions. The brain is not underactivated, as in Classic

ADHD. It is dramatically overactivated — running at a voltage and frequency that makes sensory experience overwhelming, emotional regulation nearly impossible, and behavioural control exhausting.

The Symptom Cluster

Ring of Fire ADHD presents with a characteristic and distinctive cluster: sensory hypersensitivity — the world is too loud, too bright, too textured, too fragrant, too much; emotional intensity and volatility that exceeds even the Limbic type in the speed and severity of shifts; extreme difficulty with transitions and changes in routine; pronounced mood cycles that are shorter than bipolar episodes but considerably more intense than normal mood variation; oppositional and defiant behaviour driven not by willfulness but by a nervous system that is in a state of near-constant overwhelm; difficulty filtering irrelevant stimuli at both sensory and cognitive levels; and periods of seemingly bizarre or disorganised thinking when overwhelm peaks.

Zara's experience of the fluorescent lights as genuinely painful, the difficulty with noise that others don't register, the combustible quality of her emotional responses — all are features of a brain whose excitatory-inhibitory balance is tilted dramatically toward excitation. This is not metaphorical hyperactivation. It is measurable, visible in the QEEG, and directly explicable through the glutamate/GABA dysregulation discussed in Chapter Four.

In children, Ring of Fire ADHD is among the most dramatic and distressing presentations: these are children who seem to be in a state of constant overwhelm, who erupt without apparent proportionate triggers, who cannot tolerate the sensory environment of a normal classroom, and who are frequently misdiagnosed as bipolar disorder — particularly when the emotional cycles are prominent.

In adults, years of experience managing the overwhelm produce more controlled external presentations, but at the cost of enormous ongoing cognitive effort and a chronic state of depletion.

SPECT and QEEG Findings

SPECT in Ring of Fire ADHD shows generalised increased activity across the cortex — not focal hyperperfusion as in the Overfocused type, but a diffuse pattern of cortical hyperactivation that Amen's database has associated specifically with this presentation and with its characteristic treatment resistance to stimulants (Amen, 2013). The subcortical structures, including the basal ganglia and thalamus, may also show elevated activity, contributing to the sensory gating failures that produce hypersensitivity.

QEEG shows diffuse elevated high-beta (20–35 Hz) and sometimes gamma (35 Hz and above) across multiple electrode sites, with the ring-like distribution visible on topographic maps. Alpha power is typically reduced across the cortex — the brain has minimal capacity to slow down and rest. The coherence map may show abnormal hypersynchrony in some cortical networks, suggesting a pattern of neural circuits that are excessively coupled and insufficiently able to operate independently.

This pattern is the neurophysiological opposite of Classic ADHD's theta-excess/beta-deficit signature. Where Classic ADHD shows a brain running too slowly, Ring of Fire shows a brain running far too fast. The treatment implications are consequently opposite.

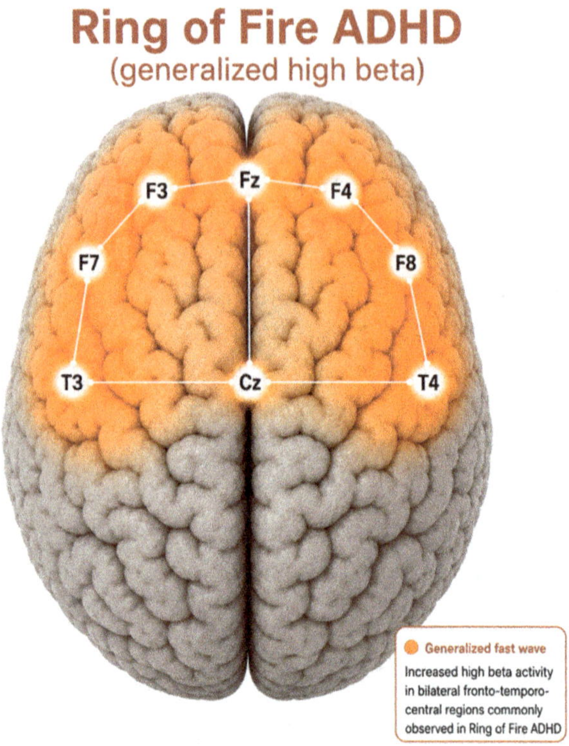

Neurochemical Profile

Ring of Fire ADHD is the presentation most clearly associated with glutamate excess and GABA deficiency in cortical circuits. The excitatory-inhibitory imbalance drives the cortical overactivation, the sensory hypersensitivity (insufficient sensory gating), and the emotional volatility (limbic circuits that are inadequately inhibited). Inflammatory cytokines — which have been shown to influence glutamate metabolism and GABA function — may contribute to the pattern in some individuals, and anti-inflammatory approaches are potentially relevant.

In some individuals with Ring of Fire ADHD, neuroinflammation may be actively sustaining the cortical overactivation rather than merely accompanying it. When the brain's immune cells — microglia — are triggered by systemic inflammation, infection, or chronic stress, they release excess glutamate into the synaptic environment while simultaneously weakening the brain's GABA-based braking system. Pro-inflammatory cytokines including TNF-α and IL-6 compound this by disrupting dopamine synthesis and amplifying excitatory signalling. The practical implication is significant: for individuals with Ring of Fire ADHD who also have a history of immune dysregulation, atopic conditions, autoimmune disorders, or chronic systemic inflammation, reducing that inflammatory load is not a complementary strategy — it is a central one.

What Ring of Fire ADHD Is Confused With

Bipolar disorder is the primary diagnostic confusion and is of considerable clinical importance because of its treatment implications. The bipolar diagnosis frequently leads to trial of mood stabilisers and/or antipsychotics; the Ring of Fire diagnosis leads to anti-inflammatory and GABA-supporting approaches, with mood stabilisers as a secondary option. The QEEG distinction — diffuse high-beta in Ring of Fire versus the more complex pattern of bipolar disorder, which may include mixed fast and slow activity — is useful but not always definitive, and careful clinical assessment of episode duration, cycling pattern, and family history remains essential.

Anxiety disorders with panic and autonomic hyperactivation share the sensory hypersensitivity and emotional volatility of Ring of Fire ADHD, and the two commonly co-occur. Treatment for both is informed by anti-arousal approaches — the distinction is that Ring of Fire has a specific cortical overactivation pattern visible on QEEG, while anxiety disorders may not always show this precise pattern.

Sensory processing disorder — a condition not formally recognised in DSM-5 but well-described in the occupational therapy literature — overlaps substantially with the sensory dimension of Ring of Fire ADHD and may co-occur with it.

Medication Implications — The Critical Caution

The single most important clinical point about Ring of Fire ADHD is that stimulant medications should be used with great caution — and in many cases avoided as a first-line approach — because they increase cortical arousal in a brain that is already dramatically overaroused. The characteristic clinical trajectory of an unrecognised Ring of Fire patient who has been prescribed stimulants is one of initial modest improvement (because some attentional symptoms respond to the dopaminergic effect) followed by escalating volatility, worsening emotional dyscontrol, increasing sensory sensitivity, and sometimes emergence of psychotic or manic features that lead to a bipolar diagnosis and further treatment complications.

Where medication is needed, GABA-supporting agents — including gabapentin, low-dose valproate, and occasionally low-dose benzodiazepines in the short term — may be more appropriate first steps. Clonidine has been used due to its central alpha agonist action. Antihistamines with antiglutamatergic properties have been used in some protocols. In children, working with an integrative psychiatrist experienced in this presentation is strongly recommended before any pharmacological intervention.

Supplements targeting the glutamate/GABA balance are the most important nutritional priority: magnesium glycinate (which blocks NMDA receptors and reduces glutamate excess), L-theanine (which increases GABA activity and promotes alpha synchrony), taurine, and GABA itself. N-acetylcysteine, which modulates glutamate release through the cystine-glutamate antiporter, has emerging evidence in bipolar disorder and may be relevant in Ring of Fire.

Diet is one of the most accessible tools to manage inflammation. The ketogenic diet has the most specific relevance here: the ketone bodies produced during ketosis directly increase GABA and reduce glutamate, addressing the excitatory-inhibitory imbalance at its neurochemical root, while also dampening microglial activation and reducing inflammatory cytokines (Jiang et al., 2022). However, for most people, the best dietary starting point remains the Mediterranean pattern — rich in omega-3 fatty acids, polyphenols, and diverse plant foods — which reduces systemic inflammation broadly without the restrictiveness or nutritional risks of elimination diets. (Greenblatt, 2017).

Neurofeedback Protocol Overview

Neurofeedback for Ring of Fire ADHD involves downtraining the elevated high-beta and gamma activity — the opposite direction from Classic ADHD protocols. The goal is to reduce cortical overactivation, increase alpha (which normalises sensory gating and provides the cortical brake that is absent in this profile), and improve the brain's capacity to regulate its own excitatory-inhibitory balance. Some practitioners use SMR training (12–15 Hz) at central sites as a gentle entry point, as SMR enhancement can improve inhibitory control without further increasing cortical excitation.

Ring of Fire is a presentation where the initial neurofeedback sessions may temporarily increase symptoms as the brain begins to reorganise — a phenomenon that requires careful patient preparation, frequent communication, and willingness to adjust the protocol rapidly. The BCIA-accredited practitioner caveat is, if anything, more important here than in other presentations.

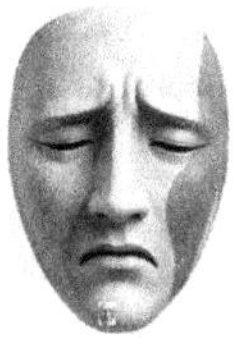

Chapter Thirteen

Type 7 — Anxious ADHD

When anxiety and attention share the same nervous system — and the treatment of one worsens the other

> ***AMIR — Age 32:*** *He arrives early. He has prepared a folder with his symptoms documented across six categories, with dates and contextual notes. He is deeply apologetic for the amount of material. He has been through three psychiatrists who diagnosed him with generalised anxiety disorder and two who diagnosed him with ADHD. He has tried four SSRIs and two stimulants. Each SSRI helped the anxiety somewhat and worsened the attention. Each stimulant helped the attention somewhat and triggered panic attacks. He is politely exhausted and quietly furious. He would like, he says, for someone to look at both problems at the same time.*

Anxious ADHD — Type 7 in Amen's framework, and a construct not formalised in DSM-5 but clinically well-established and neurophysiologically distinctive — is the type that most clearly illustrates the clinical cost of treating the symptom rather than the brain. It is the type where attention difficulties and anxiety are not merely co-occurring conditions but are intertwined at the neurophysiological level in ways that make the standard sequential approach — treat one, then treat the other — demonstrably inadequate.

Amir represents a population that is common in specialist practice: individuals who have been passed between the ADHD clinic and the anxiety clinic, each treating their piece of the presentation while the interaction between the two remains untreated. Understanding Anxious ADHD requires understanding that attention and anxiety are not separate systems that happen to malfunction simultaneously. They are interacting components of a single regulatory architecture that, in this profile, is dysregulated in ways that affect both simultaneously.

The Symptom Cluster

Anxious ADHD presents with a combination of the attentional symptoms that characterise ADHD and the physiological, cognitive, and behavioural features of anxiety — with the clinical complexity that each system amplifies the dysfunction in the other. The anxiety generates cognitive preoccupation that competes with task-directed attention, making it difficult to distinguish whether attentional failures are driven by the ADHD component or the anxiety component. The attentional difficulties, in turn, increase anxiety — missed deadlines, forgotten obligations, incomplete tasks — creating a reinforcing cycle in which each condition worsens the other.

Key features include: hypervigilance combined with attention difficulties — the paradox of a brain that is simultaneously over-attending to threats and under-attending to tasks; pervasive worry that cannot be redirected even when the person recognises its irrationality; physical symptoms of autonomic activation (rapid heart rate, gastric upset, muscle tension) that distract from cognitive tasks; a characteristic perfectionism driven by the anxiety component — extreme care in tasks that matter, combined with avoidance of tasks where performance anxiety is high; and an over-reliance on external structure and reassurance that reflects both the ADHD's difficulty with self-regulation and the anxiety's need for certainty.

The anxiety is commonly the louder presenting complaint — more distressing, more visible in consultation, more clearly connected to suffering. The ADHD dimension is often recognised only when anxiety treatment produces incomplete improvement, and the residual attentional difficulties become apparent in the absence of anxious preoccupation.

SPECT and QEEG Findings

SPECT in Anxious ADHD shows a characteristic combination: basal ganglia hyperactivation (associated with the anxious, threat-sensitive quality of the presentation) combined with prefrontal underactivation (the attentional component). The basal ganglia, including the caudate nucleus and putamen, are involved in regulating anxiety and approach-withdrawal motivation — their hyperactivation in Anxious ADHD drives the vigilant, ruminative quality of the anxiety component. The prefrontal underactivation drives the attentional difficulties and the executive function impairment.

QEEG shows a mixed pattern: elevated right frontal beta (15–20 Hz, reflecting anxious overactivation in prefrontal monitoring circuits) combined with elevated frontal theta in some cases (reflecting the underlying ADHD-related cortical underactivation). The combination of these two patterns — fast waves associated with anxious monitoring alongside slow waves associated with attentional underactivation — produces the distinctive neurophysiological signature of the anxious ADHD profile.

Coherence abnormalities, reflecting disrupted communication between prefrontal and limbic circuits, are also commonly present.

Heart rate variability (HRV) — a measure of autonomic nervous system flexibility — is typically reduced in Anxious ADHD, reflecting chronic sympathetic dominance and reduced vagal tone. HRV biofeedback, which specifically trains autonomic regulation, is a valuable complementary intervention for this profile.

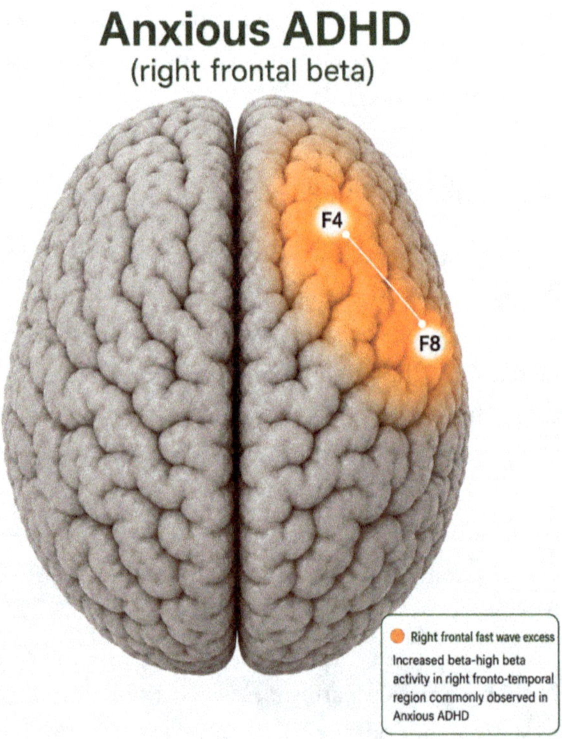

Neurochemical Profile

Anxious ADHD involves dysregulation of both the noradrenergic and dopaminergic systems — the noradrenergic component driving the hypervigilance and anxiety, the dopaminergic component driving the attentional difficulties. GABA deficiency contributes to both: insufficient GABA-ergic inhibition in prefrontal-limbic circuits allows both the anxiety circuits and the distracting DMN to run with insufficient restraint.

Glutamate excess — through mechanisms that overlap with the Ring of Fire profile but are more regionally specific, concentrated in frontal-subcortical circuits — contributes to the anxious rumination and the cognitive inflexibility that characterises worry.

What Anxious ADHD Is Confused With — and Why the Confusion Matters

Generalised anxiety disorder is the most common misdiagnosis — or incomplete diagnosis — in Anxious ADHD. The anxiety features are real, impairing, and correctly identified as warranting treatment. What is missed is the ADHD component — the attentional difficulties that are not merely secondary to the anxiety but have their own neurophysiological basis that requires separate targeting.

The consequences of treating Anxious ADHD as pure anxiety disorder are predictable: SSRIs reduce the anxious arousal somewhat but leave the attentional difficulties and executive function impairment largely unaddressed. The person feels slightly less distressed but no more able to function effectively — a partial treatment that invites the clinician to conclude that higher doses are needed, when in fact the missing intervention is one targeting the attentional component.

The consequences of treating Anxious ADHD as pure ADHD — as commonly occurs when the attentional features are prominent — are equally predictable: stimulants increase the dopaminergic drive for task engagement but also increase noradrenergic arousal, frequently worsening the anxiety, triggering panic attacks (as occurred with Amir), or producing a mixed state of improved attention and escalating anxiety that is ultimately less tolerable than either condition alone.

The correct approach requires simultaneously targeting both systems — which is precisely what an integrative, brain-based assessment using QEEG enables and a symptom-checklist approach cannot.

Medication and Supplement Implications

Medication for Anxious ADHD requires sequential or combined targeting of both components. Approaches that have been found helpful include: low-dose SSRI or SNRI to address the anxious component, combined with low-dose stimulant or non-stimulant (atomoxetine is often better tolerated in this profile than amphetamine-based stimulants, as it increases noradrenaline more selectively and has documented anxiolytic effects); clonidine or guanfacine, which reduce noradrenergic arousal and have utility in both anxiety and ADHD; and in some cases buspirone — a non-benzodiazepine anxiolytic with dopamine D2 partial agonist properties — which addresses the anxiety without further sedation and has mild attentional benefits.

Nutritional priorities include: magnesium glycinate (for GABA support and autonomous nervous system regulation); L-theanine (which increases alpha and GABA activity, promoting calm focus without sedation); ashwagandha (KSM-66 extract), which has documented cortisol-lowering and anxiolytic effects in controlled trials without impairing alertness; omega-3 EPA for mood and anxiety regulation; and inositol, particularly for the ruminative, compulsive quality of the anxiety component.

HRV biofeedback — training slow, diaphragmatic breathing at the resonant frequency of the cardiovascular system (approximately 6 breaths per minute) — is a non-pharmacological intervention with robust evidence for reducing anxiety and improving prefrontal-limbic regulatory capacity. It is one of the most accessible first-line interventions for Anxious ADHD and can be initiated immediately, alongside whatever other assessment and treatment approaches are being pursued.

Neurofeedback Protocol Overview

Neurofeedback for Anxious ADHD needs to address both the elevated frontal beta (anxiety component) and the attentional component simultaneously. Alpha enhancement protocols — training increased frontal alpha power — can accomplish both, as alpha synchrony promotes a calm, alert, attentive state that is the neurophysiological target for this presentation. SMR training at Cz (12–15 Hz), which enhances inhibitory motor and cognitive control without increasing arousal, is another well-suited approach for this profile.

The sequencing of neurofeedback in Anxious ADHD typically prioritises anxiety reduction first — partly because anxious individuals respond poorly to protocols that increase arousal before the anxiety baseline has been lowered, and partly because reducing the anxiety component often reveals more clearly the purely attentional features that can then be addressed with targeted protocols.

References — Chapters Seven through Thirteen

Amen, D.G. (2013). Healing ADD: The Breakthrough Program That Allows You to See and Heal the 7 Types of ADD (revised ed.). New York: Berkley Books.

Greenblatt, J.M. & Gottlieb, B. (2017). Finally Focused: The Breakthrough Natural Treatment Plan for ADHD. New York: Harmony Books.

Faraone, S.V. & Larsson, H. (2019). 'Genetics of attention deficit hyperactivity disorder.' Molecular Psychiatry, 24(4), 562–575.

Johnstone, J., Gunkelman, J. & Lunt, J. (2005). 'Clinical database development: characterization of EEG phenotypes.' Clinical EEG and Neuroscience, 36(2), 99–107.

Tye, C., McLoughlin, G., Kuntsi, J. & Asherson, P. (2011). 'Electrophysiological markers of genetic risk for ADHD.' Expert Reviews in Molecular Medicine, 13, e9.

Arns, M. et al. (2013). 'Evaluation of neurofeedback in ADHD: the long and winding road.' Biological Psychology, 95, 108–115.

Konofal, E. et al. (2004). 'Iron deficiency in children with attention-deficit/hyperactivity disorder.' Archives of Pediatrics and Adolescent Medicine, 158(12), 1113–1115.

Bloch, M.H. & Mulqueen, J. (2014). 'Nutritional supplements for the treatment of ADHD.' Child and Adolescent Psychiatric Clinics of North America, 23(4), 883–897.

Halmøy, A. et al. (2010). 'Plasma amino acid levels in adult attention-deficit/hyperactivity disorder.' Biological Psychiatry, 68(11), 1045–1052.

Oner, O. & Oner, P. (2015). 'Ferritin and hyperactivity ratings in attention deficit hyperactivity disorder.' *Pediatrics International*, 57(1), 57–62.

Mohammadpour, N. et al. (2018). 'Effect of vitamin D supplementation as adjunctive therapy to methylphenidate on ADHD symptoms.' *Nutritional Neuroscience*, 21(3), 202–209.

Ischebeck, M. et al. (2014). 'Frontal EEG alpha asymmetry in obsessive compulsive disorder.' *Neuropsychologia*, 65, 116–124.

Bucci, P. et al. (2004). 'Executive hypercontrol in obsessive-compulsive disorder: electrophysiological and neuropsychological indices.' *Clinical Neurophysiology*, 115(6), 1340–1348.

Bhatt, R.R. et al. (2015). 'Frontal EEG alpha activity and obsessive-compulsive behaviors in non-clinical young adults: a pilot study.' *Frontiers in Psychology*, 6, 1480.

Cortese, S. et al. (2016). 'Neurofeedback for ADHD: meta-analysis of clinical and neuropsychological outcomes from randomised controlled trials.' Journal of the American Academy of Child & Adolescent Psychiatry, 55(6), 444–455.

Micoulaud-Franchi, J.A. et al. (2014). 'EEG neurofeedback treatments in children with ADHD: an updated meta-analysis of randomised controlled trials.' Frontiers in Human Neuroscience, 8, 906.

Gevensleben, H. et al. (2009). 'Is neurofeedback an efficacious treatment for ADHD? A randomised controlled clinical trial.' Journal of Child Psychology and Psychiatry, 50(7), 780–789.

van Dongen-Boomsma, M. et al. (2013). 'A randomised placebo-controlled trial of EEG neurofeedback in children with ADHD.' Journal of Clinical Psychiatry, 74(8), 821–827.

Lubar, J.F. & Shouse, M.N. (1976). 'EEG and behavioral changes in a hyperkinetic child concurrent with training of the sensorimotor rhythm (SMR).' Biofeedback and Self-Regulation, 1(3), 293–306.

Leins, U. et al. (2007). 'Neurofeedback for children with ADHD: a comparison of SCP and theta/beta protocols.' Applied Psychophysiology and Biofeedback, 32(2), 73–88.

Duric, N.S. et al. (2012). 'Neurofeedback for the treatment of children and adolescents with ADHD.' Journal of Child and Adolescent Psychopharmacology, 22(1), 19–28.

Rossiter, T. (2004). 'The effectiveness of neurofeedback and stimulant drugs in treating AD/HD.' Applied Psychophysiology and Biofeedback, 29(2), 95–112.

Ros, T. et al. (2014). 'Consensus on the reporting and experimental design of clinical and cognitive-behavioural neurofeedback studies.' Brain Topography, 27(1), 74–87.

Lofthouse, N. et al. (2012). 'A review of neurofeedback treatment for pediatric ADHD.' Journal of Attention Disorders, 16(5), 351–372.

Sonuga-Barke, E.J.S. et al. (2013). 'Nonpharmacological interventions for ADHD: systematic review and meta-analyses of randomised controlled trials.' American Journal of Psychiatry, 170(3), 275–289.

Monastra, V.J. et al. (2005). 'Electroencephalographic biofeedback in the treatment of ADHD.' Applied Psychophysiology and Biofeedback, 30(2), 95–114.

Bridge to Part Three

FROM THE BRAIN TO THE TREATMENT PLAN

Seven brains. Seven different patterns of electrical activity, metabolic function, and neurochemical balance. Seven different clinical presentations that share a diagnostic label without sharing an aetiology. Seven different treatment approaches — different medications, different supplements, different neurofeedback protocols, different starting priorities.

Part Two has shown what becomes visible when we look at the brain rather than the behaviour. The QEEG and SPECT findings for each subtype are not merely academic correlates of clinical presentations. They are the biological basis for treatment decisions that the symptom checklist cannot support. They are the reason why Zara's improvement depends on protocols that are precisely opposite to Liam's. They are why Oliver's rigidity gets worse on the medication that helps Liam's impulsivity. They are why Maya's antidepressants produce partial relief without resolution.

Part Three builds directly on the subtype framework established here. We will examine the problems with current pharmacological approaches — the tolerance, the side effects, the long-term consequences — with greater depth than Chapter Five allowed, and then offer the integrative treatment model that the seven subtypes demand: functional laboratory testing, dietary foundations, lifestyle interventions, targeted supplementation specific to each neurobiological profile, neurofeedback, and — when medication is genuinely indicated — the use of pharmacological tools guided by neurophysiological data rather than by symptom category alone.

The goal is not to replace medication with supplements, or to replace psychiatry with neurofeedback. The goal is to build a treatment approach in which every intervention is selected on the basis of what that specific brain needs — measured, not guessed; targeted, not generic; monitored over time, not assumed to be working because the rating scale hasn't gotten worse.

Liam's brain deserves better than what it has received. So do Priya's, Oliver's, Zara's, Daniel's, and Maya's. Part Three is where we begin to show what better looks like.

PART THREE
Beyond the Prescription Pad

If Parts One and Two have done their job, you arrive here with a different set of questions than most ADHD books generate. Not 'which medication should I be on?' but 'which type of brain am I, and what does that brain need?' Not 'why won't my child behave?' but 'what is happening neurologically, and what would genuinely help?' Not 'how do I manage my symptoms?' but 'how do I build the conditions under which my brain can genuinely thrive?'

These are better questions. They are harder to answer — because they require more than a prescription and a follow-up in six weeks. They require understanding the brain, the body, the gut, the hormones, the sleep architecture, the nutritional environment, the digital habits, and the unique vulnerabilities of each neurobiological subtype. They require, in short, the approach that functional and integrative psychiatry exists to provide.

Part Three is the practical half of this book. Each chapter addresses a different domain of the integrative treatment model, with the specific application to ADHD subtypes made explicit throughout. Each chapter closes with an Action Plan — a set of concrete, implementable steps that can be started this week, not after a specialist referral that takes six months.

We begin where every honest discussion of ADHD treatment must begin: with what current approaches do well, what they don't, and what has to change.

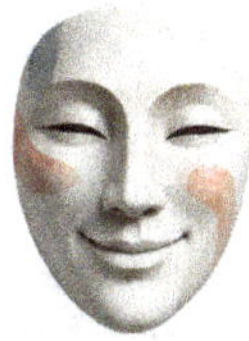

Chapter Fourteen

What Works, What Doesn't, and What We're Missing

An honest appraisal of medications, therapy, and the gap between them

> ***LIAM — Age 25, Post-Assessment:*** *His QEEG shows exactly what the literature predicts for Classic ADHD. His psychiatrist explains that the medication he was prescribed at age ten was probably the right first choice for his neurotype — and that the problem was never the medication, but what surrounded it. No dietary assessment. No sleep evaluation. No neurofeedback. No functional testing. No acknowledgement that the medication was a starting point, not a destination. Liam has been on medication for fifteen years and has received almost nothing else. He is not surprised. He is exhausted by it.*

Let us begin with what is true.

Stimulant medications work. For the right neurobiological profile — particularly Classic and some Inattentive presentations — methylphenidate and amphetamine-based medications produce short-term improvements in sustained attention, impulse control, and behavioural regulation that are genuine, measurable, and often transformative. Effect sizes in short-term controlled trials are among the largest in psychiatry. For a child who has spent years failing in school, for an adult who has never experienced a full working day of productive focus, the first weeks of effective stimulant treatment can feel like an extraordinary relief. That relief is not illusory.

This book is not anti-medication. It never has been. Medications for ADHD, used appropriately and for the right neurobiological profile, are valuable tools that help real people. Any book that suggests otherwise is doing its readers a disservice.

What this chapter is about is the gap between what medications are and what they have been positioned as. The difference between a useful tool and the complete treatment. The difference between short-term symptom relief and the long-term brain health that every person with ADHD deserves.

What Medications Do Well

Stimulant medications act on the dopaminergic and noradrenergic systems to produce rapid improvements in attentional regulation, impulse inhibition, and — in the right profiles — emotional modulation. For Classic ADHD, methylphenidate measurably normalises the theta/beta ratio within hours of administration — primarily by increasing beta power in frontal regions — and produces concurrent improvements in CPT performance on objective attentional measures. This effect was documented in landmark Australian research conducted in Sydney, where Clarke, Barry, McCarthy, and Selikowitz demonstrated that EEG patterns predict methylphenidate response and that stimulant medications produce measurable electrophysiological changes in children with ADHD (Clarke et al., 2002; Clarke et al., 2003; Clarke et al., 2017). These are not placebo effects. They are neurophysiological changes, visible in QEEG, that correspond to the clinical improvement patients and teachers report.

For children and adults in whom the diagnostic profile is clear, the neurobiological subtype is appropriate for stimulant treatment, and the short-term goals include enabling educational engagement, reducing dangerous impulsivity, or restoring basic occupational functioning, medication is an important and evidence-backed intervention. The effect sizes for short-term symptom reduction are real. The speed of onset — often visible within the first dose — is clinically valuable when the situation is urgent.

Non-stimulant medications add to the toolkit usefully. Atomoxetine's specific noradrenergic mechanism makes it better suited than stimulants for certain presentations, particularly Anxious ADHD and individuals in whom stimulant side effects are limiting. Guanfacine and clonidine offer prefrontal-enhancing and anxiety-reducing effects through alpha-2 adrenergic agonism, with particular utility in children with significant emotional dysregulation. Bupropion's combined dopaminergic and noradrenergic action suits the Limbic presentation that also needs mood support. These are legitimate pharmacological tools with important roles in the integrative treatment plan.

Cognitive-behavioural therapy (CBT) for ADHD, while not addressing the underlying neurobiology, provides the scaffolding of compensatory strategies — organisation systems, time management tools, behavioural routines — that help many individuals bridge the gap between their neurological limitations and the demands of their environment. For adults particularly, structured CBT targeting executive function has a good evidence base that extends the benefit of medication or supplements. Motivational interviewing, acceptance-based approaches, and

ADHD coaching offer additional layers of support. These are valuable contributions.

What Medications Don't Do

Medications suppress symptoms. They do not alter the underlying neurobiology that generates those symptoms. This is not a criticism unique to ADHD medications — most psychiatric pharmacology works this way. But it has specific implications that are rarely communicated clearly to patients.

When methylphenidate is discontinued, symptoms return to baseline. This is not a failure of the medication; it is a description of its mechanism. Medications for ADHD are not *neuroplastic* interventions. They do not train the brain to regulate itself more effectively. They do not build the prefrontal circuitry whose delayed development drives so much of the Classic ADHD presentation. They provide a daily chemical override of a regulatory system that is not functioning optimally — an override that stops working when the override is removed. This is why, as documented in Chapter Five, the long-term functional outcomes of medication-only treatment are considerably weaker than the short-term symptom data would lead one to expect.

The tolerance problem, also established in Chapter Five, is the pharmacological expression of this: the brain, encountering a daily bolus of dopaminergic stimulation, adapts by upregulating the dopamine transporter and reducing receptor sensitivity — meaning that the medication progressively works against its own mechanism. The dose required to maintain the original effect climbs. The window of effectiveness narrows. For many patients, the trajectory over years is dose escalation followed by loss of effect followed by medication change followed by the same cycle on a different molecule. This is not optimal management. It is, in many cases, what happens when symptom suppression is the only treatment strategy in use.

Talk therapy, for all its genuine value in building compensatory strategies, does not change the QEEG. A person with Classic ADHD who has excellent CBT skills and comprehensive organisational systems still has a frontal theta excess pattern that drives their underlying neurological vulnerabilities. The skills help them manage those vulnerabilities more effectively; they do not reduce the vulnerability itself. This distinction matters for setting realistic expectations and for understanding why strategies alone, without addressing the underlying neurobiology, rarely feel like enough.

What Is Missing — and What Part Three Provides

The treatment gap in ADHD is not primarily a gap in pharmacological tools. It is a gap in breadth: the absence of systematic attention to the nutritional, metabolic, hormonal, gastrointestinal, sleep, and lifestyle factors that determine how well any brain — ADHD or otherwise — can regulate itself, and that in ADHD brains carry disproportionate clinical weight.

A child on methylphenidate whose ferritin is 14 ng/mL is on a medication that is working against an iron-deficient dopamine synthesis system. The medication is not failing them. But the nutritional environment in which it is operating is substantially limiting its effectiveness — and addressing the iron deficiency might reduce the dose required, improve the response, or in some cases resolve the attentional difficulties without continued medication. This child is not unusual. They are common. And the iron is almost never checked.

An adult with Anxious ADHD whose gut microbiome is depleted, whose sleep is consistently under six hours, whose magnesium levels are in the low-normal range, who is on a diet high in refined carbohydrates and low in omega-3 fatty acids — this person's neurological environment is actively working against their brain's regulatory capacity on multiple fronts simultaneously. Adding an SNRI to this environment is not futile, but it is insufficient. The integrative model addresses all of these factors, in a sequence and combination calibrated to the specific subtype.

The chapters that follow address each domain in turn: diet and nutrigenomics, gut health, sleep, exercise, subtype-specific supplementation, digital environment, neurofeedback and mindfulness, women's hormones, and finally the practical strategies for work and study. Each ends with a specific action plan. Together, they constitute not a replacement for medical care but a framework for the medical care that ADHD deserves.

A Note on Functional Testing

Before addressing each domain, a word about the foundation: functional laboratory testing. The integrative approach to ADHD is not about adding supplements on top of standard care. It is about identifying the specific biological vulnerabilities of the individual — and the first step in that identification is measurement.

A minimum functional testing panel for anyone pursuing an integrative ADHD assessment should include: full blood count and iron studies including ferritin (not just haemoglobin — serum ferritin below 30 ng/mL is functionally significant for brain health even in the absence of clinical anaemia); zinc and copper levels (with calculation of the zinc/copper ratio, discussed in the next chapter); serum 25-hydroxyvitamin D; thyroid function including TSH, free T4, and free T3; comprehensive metabolic panel; red blood cell magnesium (which reflects tissue stores more accurately than serum magnesium); fasting homocysteine (a sensitive marker of methylation capacity and B12/folate adequacy); B12 and folate levels; and MTHFR and COMT genetic variant analysis where available.

Additionally, a comprehensive stool analysis assessing microbiome diversity, short-chain fatty acid production, intestinal permeability markers, and inflammatory markers provides the gut health foundation discussed in Chapter Sixteen. In some cases, organic acid testing and amino acid profiling add important information about neurotransmitter metabolite patterns. This is not an exhaustive list; clinical judgment determines which tests are most relevant for each individual's presentation and history.

Testing is not the end of assessment — it is the beginning of targeted intervention. What follows in the coming chapters is built on the assumption that we are working with specific, measured data about a specific individual's biology, rather than applying generic protocols to a diagnostic category.

✦ Action Plan — Chapter Fourteen

→ Request a functional testing panel from your GP or integrative practitioner. At minimum: ferritin, zinc, copper, vitamin D (25-OH), fasting homocysteine, B12, folate, thyroid function (TSH, free T4, free T3), red blood cell magnesium, and a lipid panel.

→ Ask for MTHFR and COMT genetic variant testing — these are available through standard pathology in most countries and have direct implications for nutritional supplementation strategy.

→ Document your current medication, dose, timing, and your subjective rating of its effectiveness over the past four weeks on a scale of 1–10. This baseline will allow objective comparison as integrative interventions are added.

→ If you are on stimulant medication, discuss with your prescriber whether a medication break (a structured drug holiday during holidays or leave) can provide useful information about your current baseline functioning and the extent of any tolerance development.

→ Make a list of the domains you most want to improve — attention, impulsivity, mood, sleep, emotional regulation, anxiety — in order of priority. This list will guide which chapters are most immediately relevant to your situation.

References — Chapter Fourteen

Clarke, A.R., Barry, R.J., McCarthy, R. & Selikowitz, M. (2002). 'EEG differences between good and poor responders to methylphenidate and dexamphetamine in children with attention-deficit/hyperactivity disorder.' *Clinical Neurophysiology*, 113(2), 194–205.

Clarke, A.R., Barry, R.J., McCarthy, R., Selikowitz, M., Clarke, D.C. & Croft, R.J. (2003). 'Effects of stimulant medications on children with attention-deficit/hyperactivity disorder and excessive beta activity in their EEG.' *Clinical Neurophysiology*, 114(9), 1729–1737.

Clarke, A.R., Barry, R.J., Baker, I.E., McCarthy, R. & Selikowitz, M. (2017). 'An investigation of stimulant effects on the EEG of children with attention-deficit/hyperactivity disorder.' *Clinical EEG and Neuroscience*, 48(4), 235–242.

Cortese, S. et al. (2018). 'Comparative efficacy and tolerability of medications for attention-deficit hyperactivity disorder in children, adolescents, and adults: a systematic review and network meta-analysis.' The Lancet Psychiatry, 5(9), 727–738.

Safren, S.A. et al. (2010). 'Cognitive-behavioral therapy vs relaxation with educational support for medication-treated adults with ADHD and persistent symptoms.' JAMA, 304(8), 875–880.

Solanto, M.V. et al. (2010). 'Efficacy of meta-cognitive therapy for adult ADHD.' American Journal of Psychiatry, 167(8), 958–968.

Faraone, S.V. et al. (2021). 'The World Federation of ADHD International Consensus Statement: 208 evidence-based conclusions about the disorder.' Neuroscience & Biobehavioral Reviews, 128, 789–818.

Wigal, T. et al. (2011). 'Efficacy and safety limitations of attention-deficit hyperactivity disorder pharmacotherapy in children and adults.' CNS Drugs, 25(S1), 1–12.

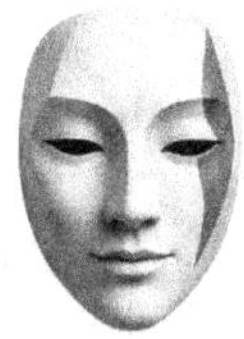

Chapter Fifteen
You Are What Your Genes Can Process

Diet, nutrigenomics, and the modifiable genetics of the ADHD brain

> ***MAYA — Age 38:*** *Her homocysteine came back at 18.4 μmol/L. The reference range says anything below 15 is normal. Her GP said it was 'a little high' and suggested she drink more water. Her integrative psychiatrist looks at it differently: at 18.4, Maya's methylation cycle is struggling. Her serotonin synthesis is likely impaired. Her dopamine recycling is compromised. Her B12 and folate are technically within range but at the lower end. She has the MTHFR C677T variant — one copy. This explains a great deal. It also, for the first time, gives her a place to start.*

Nutrigenomics is a word that sounds more exotic than it is. It means, simply: the study of how your genetic variants determine how you process nutrients — and how those nutrients in turn determine which of your genes are expressed, and how actively. In the context of ADHD, it is one of the most clinically important and most consistently overlooked areas of assessment.

The ADHD brain is not metabolically average. It has specific nutritional dependencies — requirements for cofactors in neurotransmitter synthesis, enzyme function, and neural membrane maintenance — that are elevated compared to neurotypical brains. It also carries, in many cases, genetic variants that compromise its ability to process those nutrients effectively even when they are nominally available. The result is a brain that is often operating with a nutritional handicap that no amount of effort, medication, or therapy can compensate for — but that a targeted dietary and supplementation approach can meaningfully address.

MTHFR — The Methylation Gene That Changes Everything

MTHFR — methylenetetrahydrofolate reductase — is an enzyme responsible for converting folate from food into methylfolate, the active form that the brain uses to methylate neurotransmitters. 'Methylation' refers to the addition of a methyl group (one carbon and three hydrogen atoms) to a molecule — a process that activates or deactivates enzymes, regulates gene expression, converts one neurotransmitter to another, and maintains the integrity of DNA. Without adequate methylation, the synthesis and recycling of serotonin, dopamine, and noradrenaline is compromised at the most fundamental biochemical level.

The MTHFR gene has two clinically significant variants: C677T and A1298C. Carrying one copy of C677T (heterozygous) reduces MTHFR enzyme function by approximately 30–40%. Carrying two copies (homozygous) reduces it by 60–70%. Carrying one copy of each variant compounds the effect. Approximately 10–15% of the population carries two copies of C677T; approximately 40% carry at least one copy of either variant. The relationship between MTHFR variants and ADHD is an area of active research with findings that are suggestive but not yet definitive. The most important qualification is that the two variants behave differently.

The A1298C polymorphism has the stronger and more consistent association with ADHD specifically: a 2022 meta-analysis found A1298C to be significantly associated with ADHD, and individual studies have found the hetero-homozygous A1298C genotype significantly overrepresented in ADHD children compared to controls, across both sexes (Gokcen et al., 2018). The C677T variant — more commonly discussed in popular MTHFR literature — shows a less consistent ADHD-specific association; in some studies, the heterozygous C677T genotype actually appears at lower rates in ADHD populations than controls, a finding interpreted as a heterozygous advantage rather than a risk factor. C677T's strongest psychiatric associations are with schizophrenia and bipolar disorder rather than ADHD, where the homozygous TT genotype — which reduces enzyme function by approximately 75% — carries the greatest risk.

More broadly, impaired methylation through either variant has been associated across the psychiatric spectrum: depression, bipolar disorder, schizophrenia, autism, and ADHD all show enrichment for MTHFR variants compared to the general population, consistent with the central role of methylation in neurotransmitter synthesis across neurological presentations (Wan et al., 2022). The clinical implication for practice is therefore not to test for MTHFR as a diagnostic tool for ADHD, but to test for it as a modifiable neurochemical vulnerability.

The clinical consequence of MTHFR impairment is elevated homocysteine — because the methylation cycle that would normally clear homocysteine is running below capacity. Elevated homocysteine (above 10 µmol/L, and certainly above 15 µmol/L) is associated with impaired cognitive function, mood dysregulation, vascular inflammation, and reduced neurotransmitter synthesis efficiency. It is a measurable, correctable biomarker of a modifiable neurochemical vulnerability.

The intervention is straightforward and effective: rather than standard folic acid supplementation (which requires conversion by the impaired MTHFR enzyme), supplementation with methylfolate (5-methyltetrahydrofolate, 5-MTHF) bypasses the impaired step entirely. Combined with methylcobalamin (the active, methylated form of B12), methylfolate directly supports the methylation cycle, reduces homocysteine, and improves the neurochemical environment for neurotransmitter synthesis. For individuals with MTHFR variants, this is not optional nutritional enhancement. It is correction of a biochemical impairment that is driving their neurological presentation. Maya's elevated homocysteine, her MTHFR heterozygosity, and her partial response to antidepressants fit this pattern precisely. The methylfolate intervention is not a replacement for her other treatment; it is the nutritional foundation on which everything else can work more effectively.

COMT — The Gene That Determines How Long Dopamine Lasts

COMT — catechol-O-methyltransferase — encodes an enzyme responsible for degrading dopamine and noradrenaline in the prefrontal cortex. The COMT Val158Met polymorphism is one of the most studied genetic variants in psychiatric research: the Val/Val variant produces a more active enzyme that clears dopamine rapidly, resulting in lower prefrontal dopamine availability. The Met/Met variant produces a slower enzyme, resulting in higher prefrontal dopamine but potentially greater dopamine receptor downregulation under stress.

The COMT Val/Val variant — commonly called the 'warrior' genotype — is associated with lower baseline prefrontal dopamine and consequently better performance under stress (because the lower baseline means there is more room for dopamine to rise). In everyday low-stress conditions, however, Val/Val individuals have relatively reduced prefrontal dopamine and consequently greater vulnerability to attentional difficulties. The Met/Met variant — the 'worrier' genotype — has higher baseline prefrontal dopamine, better baseline cognitive performance, but greater vulnerability to dopamine overflow under stress, which can produce cognitive disorganisation and the anxiety-cognitive interaction described in Chapter Thirteen.

COMT genotype has direct implications for treatment. Val/Val individuals have greater relative benefit from interventions that increase dopamine availability — including stimulant medications, L-tyrosine supplementation, and dopaminergic dietary patterns. Met/Met individuals may respond more sensitively to stimulants (requiring lower doses) and may benefit more from COMT-supporting interventions — including magnesium, which slows COMT activity, and catechol-containing foods like green tea — that slow dopamine clearance rather than increasing its production.

The clinical implication is that COMT genotyping, combined with MTHFR status, provides a meaningful pharmacogenomic framework for ADHD treatment — informing not just which supplements are most relevant but also which medication approach is most likely to be effective and well-tolerated. This is not speculative pharmacogenomics. It is the direct application of well-established molecular biology to clinical decision-making.

Zinc and Copper — The Balance That Modern Soil Has Disturbed

Zinc occupies a central position in ADHD neurobiology that is disproportionate to the attention it receives in standard clinical practice. It is a cofactor in dopamine synthesis, essential for the function of the dopamine transporter, required for adequate melatonin production, involved in GABA receptor function, and a modulator of both glutamate and serotonin activity. Deficiency in any of these domains produces neurological consequences; zinc deficiency, affecting all of them simultaneously, produces a neurological environment that is specifically hostile to the regulatory functions that ADHD brains are already struggling to maintain.

The challenge is that zinc deficiency has become remarkably common in ways that are invisible to standard clinical testing. Modern intensive agricultural practices have progressively depleted the zinc content of soil — and consequently of the food grown in it. A tomato grown in zinc-depleted soil contains a fraction of the zinc of the same variety grown fifty years ago. Meat from animals raised on zinc-depleted pasture is similarly affected. The result is a population-level decline in dietary zinc availability that is not reflected in any standard blood test ordered by a GP, and that is disproportionately affecting the neurologically vulnerable.

Standard serum zinc testing, moreover, is an unreliable measure of zinc adequacy, because the body maintains serum zinc within a narrow range even as intracellular and tissue stores are depleted. Compounding this, laboratory reference ranges for serum zinc have shifted progressively downward over decades, a phenomenon that reflects not improved precision but the statistical reality that reference ranges are derived from population norms — and as zinc deficiency has become more prevalent across the general population due to soil depletion and dietary change, the 'normal' range has quietly recalibrated itself around a population that is, on average, less zinc-replete than it once was. A result reported as 'normal' today may represent a level that would have been flagged as borderline deficient a generation ago. Red blood cell zinc and hair mineral analysis provide more meaningful information about actual zinc status, though both require interpretation by a practitioner familiar with the methodology.

The copper balance is equally important. Zinc and copper compete for absorption and for binding sites on key proteins. Excess copper — which is common in the context of zinc deficiency, because the competitive relationship means that as zinc declines, copper accumulates — is directly neurotoxic at elevated levels and is associated with anxiety, paranoia, and the emotional volatility that characterises several ADHD subtypes. The zinc/copper ratio (measured as serum zinc divided by serum copper) provides a clinically useful index: a ratio below 0.8 suggests relative copper excess, and is associated with increased neurological and behavioural symptoms in several studies (Walsh, 2012).

Zinc supplementation (typically 15–30 mg of zinc glycinate or zinc picolinate daily, for its superior absorption) simultaneously corrects zinc deficiency and helps normalise the zinc/copper ratio. Several randomised controlled trials have found that zinc supplementation reduces ADHD symptom severity, reduces the dose of stimulant medication required for symptom control, and improves the TOVA attentional performance in deficient children (Bilici et al., 2004; Akhondzadeh et al., 2004). Effect sizes are not large enough to replace medication. But they are clinically meaningful contributions to the neurochemical environment.

Iron and Ferritin — The Silent Driver

Iron deficiency is the most common nutritional deficiency in the world, and among the most consistently documented nutritional correlates of ADHD severity. The relationship is not surprising: iron is a required cofactor for the enzyme tyrosine hydroxylase, which catalyses the rate-limiting step in dopamine synthesis. Without adequate iron, the dopamine synthesis chain is bottlenecked at its first step — no amount of tyrosine, the amino acid precursor, will produce adequate dopamine if the enzyme that converts it is iron-dependent and iron is scarce.

The critical clinical point is that iron deficiency of neurological consequence precedes clinical anaemia by months or years. Ferritin — the iron storage protein — declines progressively as the body's iron reserves deplete, before haemoglobin and red blood cell indices are affected. At ferritin levels below 30 ng/mL — levels that are entirely within the 'normal' reference range used by most laboratories, whose lower limits are typically 10–15 ng/mL — attentional performance, sleep quality, and dopaminergic function are already measurably impaired. At ferritin below 20 ng/mL, the impairment is clinically significant. Many children and adults with ADHD presenting to general practitioners have ferritin in the 12–25 ng/mL range and are told their iron is 'normal.'

Multiple studies have found that children with ADHD have significantly lower ferritin levels than age-matched controls, and that ferritin level correlates inversely with ADHD symptom severity — more iron deficient means more severely symptomatic (Konofal et al., 2004; Cortese et al., 2012). Iron supplementation in iron-deficient children with ADHD produces improvements in ADHD rating scores that are not as rapid as stimulant medication but are sustained, measurable, and achieved without Schedule II controlled substances. For children with ferritin below 30 ng/mL, iron supplementation should arguably be the first intervention, preceding medication — a sequence that almost never happens in standard clinical practice.

Vitamin D — The Hormone That Everyone Is Deficient In

Vitamin D is technically a hormone — produced in the skin upon ultraviolet B exposure and converted in the liver and kidneys to its active form, 1,25-dihydroxycholecalciferol or calcitriol. Its receptors are distributed throughout the brain, with particularly high density in regions involved in dopamine production (the substantia nigra and ventral tegmental area) and in the prefrontal cortex. Vitamin D regulates the expression of enzymes involved in dopamine and serotonin synthesis, modulates neuroinflammatory processes, and supports neuroplasticity through effects on brain-derived neurotrophic factor (BDNF) expression.

Vitamin D deficiency is endemic — estimated to affect more than 40% of the global population, with significantly higher prevalence in higher latitudes, in individuals who work indoors, in people with darker skin pigmentation (who require longer UV exposure to produce equivalent vitamin D), and in those who apply sunscreen consistently — an increasingly common practice that, while important for skin cancer prevention, blocks up to 95–98% of the UVB radiation required for cutaneous vitamin D synthesis and has contributed meaningfully to population-level deficiency even in sun-rich climates. In ADHD populations, multiple studies have found lower 25-hydroxyvitamin D levels than in matched controls, and several randomised trials have found that vitamin D supplementation improves ADHD symptom ratings in deficient individuals (Mohammadpour et al., 2018).

Target 25-hydroxyvitamin D for optimal neurological function is 75–125 nmol/L (30–50 ng/mL) — a level that the majority of the population does not achieve through diet and sun exposure alone, particularly in temperate climates. It is worth noting that the standard 1000 IU vitamin D3 supplement commonly available over the counter is frequently inadequate for correcting established deficiency — particularly when taken for short periods. Repleting a significantly depleted individual requires higher doses sustained over months, and the common clinical error is to prescribe a modest dose briefly, retest too early, find modest improvement, and conclude that supplementation is working adequately when the target range has not been approached. Supplementation with 2000–5000 IU of vitamin D3 daily is appropriate for most individuals who test deficient and safe for long-term use at these doses, ideally combined with vitamin K2 in its most bioavailable form — menaquinone-7 (MK-7), the long-chain activated form that remains in circulation significantly longer than the shorter-chain MK-4 found in many cheaper preparations. K2 as MK-7 activates the proteins osteocalcin and matrix Gla-protein, which direct calcium toward bone mineralisation and away from arterial walls and soft tissue — an important consideration when supplementing vitamin D at doses sufficient to meaningfully increase calcium absorption. A dose of 100–200 µg of MK-7 daily is appropriate alongside vitamin D3 supplementation at these levels, taken with a fat-containing meal as both are fat-soluble vitamins whose absorption depends on dietary fat.

B12, Folate, and the Methylation Network

Vitamin B12 and folate work in concert within the methylation cycle — B12 as methylcobalamin accepting the methyl group from methylfolate and donating it to homocysteine (converting it to methionine), and folate regenerating the methyl group to continue the cycle. Both deficiencies produce elevated homocysteine. Both impair neurotransmitter synthesis. Both are extraordinarily common, particularly in populations following plant-based diets (B12 is found almost exclusively in animal products), in individuals with low stomach acid or taking proton pump inhibitors (which reduce B12 absorption), and in those with MTHFR variants (who cannot activate standard folic acid).

Testing should include both B12 and folate serum levels, plus homocysteine as a functional indicator of methylation adequacy. A B12 in the low-normal range (below 400 pmol/L) with elevated homocysteine is clinically meaningful even if the laboratory reference range calls it 'normal.' Supplementation should use the active forms — methylcobalamin for B12 (not cyanocobalamin, which requires additional metabolic conversion), and methylfolate for folate (not folic acid, which is improperly processed by MTHFR-variant individuals).

The dietary approach to supporting methylation includes: dark leafy vegetables — raw or lightly steamed (spinach, broccoli, Brussels sprouts) for natural folate; eggs, animal proteins and fermented dairy (yoghurt, kefir) for B12; and avoidance of processed foods containing synthetic folic acid — which, in individuals with MTHFR variants, can accumulate unconverted and paradoxically block methylfolate receptors in the brain.

Lithium — The Overlooked Trace Mineral

Lithium, in the pharmacological doses used for bipolar disorder, is a mood stabiliser with a well-established evidence base. In trace doses — lithium orotate or lithium carbonate at 1–5 mg daily, as opposed to the 300–1200 mg used therapeutically — it is a naturally occurring trace mineral found in drinking water and soil, with documented neurological functions including supporting BDNF — the brain fertilizer, neuroprotective effects, and modulation of glutamate activity through effects on the inositol signalling pathway.

Epidemiological studies have found inverse relationships between lithium levels in drinking water and rates of suicide, violent crime, and neurodevelopmental disorders — suggesting that population-level trace lithium availability has neurological consequences that have gone largely unrecognised in the ADHD literature. For individuals with Ring of Fire, Temporal Lobe, and Limbic subtypes — where mood instability, glutamate excess, and emotional volatility are central features — trace lithium is a rational consideration that is neither the pharmacological intervention of mood disorder treatment nor a nutritional afterthought (Schrauzer & Shrestha, 1990).

Trace lithium supplementation as lithium orotate (which crosses the blood brain barrier more effectively than carbonate) at 1–5 mg daily is safe, well-tolerated, and available over the counter in most countries. It does not require the monitoring associated with therapeutic lithium doses (thyroid function, renal function, serum levels) at these micro-doses. For clinicians and patients interested in pursuing this avenue, discussing it with a practitioner familiar with integrative approaches is appropriate — it is not a first-line intervention for most presentations, but for the emotionally volatile, glutamate-driven subtypes it represents an evidence-informed option.

The Dietary Framework — What to Eat for an ADHD Brain

No specific 'ADHD diet' has been definitively validated in large randomised trials. What has been consistently found, across nutritional psychiatry research and ADHD-specific studies, is that the same dietary patterns that support cardiovascular health and reduce systemic inflammation also support brain health and reduce ADHD symptom severity — and that the dietary patterns characteristic of modern ultra-processed food culture reliably make things worse.

The foundations are simple: a diet high in whole foods (vegetables, fruits, legumes, whole grains, nuts, seeds), quality protein sources (eggs, fish, lean meat, tofu), and fatty fish or omega-3-rich foods, while minimising ultra-processed foods, refined sugars, artificial food colours, and seed oils high in omega-6 fatty acids. The specific nutritional targets for ADHD — iron, zinc, magnesium, B12, folate, omega-3s, vitamin D — are best addressed through both food and targeted supplementation, since food sources alone are rarely sufficient given modern dietary patterns and soil depletion.

The evidence for dietary patterns in ADHD symptom severity is most robust for: omega-3 supplementation (consistent modest positive effects across multiple RCTs); elimination of artificial food colours and sodium benzoate (the McCann et al., 2007 Southampton study demonstrated measurable increases in hyperactive behaviour after challenge with artificial colours in both ADHD and non-ADHD children, leading to regulatory action in the UK); and the Mediterranean dietary pattern overall, which has been associated with reduced ADHD prevalence in cross-sectional studies and improved executive function in intervention studies.

Blood sugar regulation deserves special mention. The ADHD brain is particularly sensitive to glycaemic fluctuation — the sharp rise and subsequent crash in blood glucose that follows high-glycaemic meals produces transient neurological disruption that compounds the pre-existing attentional instability. Practical measures include: never missing breakfast; including protein in every meal; minimising refined carbohydrate and sugar consumption; choosing low-glycaemic-index grains; and having protein-containing snacks available during the day rather than relying on sustained focus in the hypoglycaemic window between meals.

✦ Action Plan — Chapter Fifteen

→ Request MTHFR and COMT genotyping alongside your functional panel. If MTHFR variants are found, switch immediately to methylfolate (5-MTHF, 400–800 µg) and methylcobalamin (1000 µg) rather than standard folic acid and cyanocobalamin.

→ Test serum ferritin (not just haemoglobin). If ferritin is below 30 ng/mL, discuss iron supplementation with your practitioner — iron bisglycinate 25–

50 mg is generally well-absorbed and gentler on the GI tract than ferrous sulphate.

→ Test serum zinc and copper. If the zinc/copper ratio is below 0.8, begin zinc glycinate 15–25 mg daily with food (not simultaneously with iron, as they compete for absorption). Take at a different meal.

→ Test 25-hydroxyvitamin D. If below 75 nmol/L, supplement with 2000–5000 IU vitamin D3 daily with a meal containing fat (as it is fat-soluble). Add vitamin K2 (100–200 µg MK-7 form) if supplementing at the higher end.

→ Test fasting homocysteine. If above 10 µmol/L, begin methylfolate (1–5 mg), methylcobalamin (1000 µg), and pyridoxal-5-phosphate (25–50 mg, the active B6 form). Retest in 3 months.

→ Restructure meals around blood sugar stability: protein and fat with every meal, breakfast within 60 minutes of waking, avoid processed carbohydrates as snacks, include protein-rich snacks mid-morning and mid-afternoon.

→ Reduce artificial food colours, sodium benzoate, and ultra-processed foods. Read labels of anything in a packet. Increase fatty fish (salmon, sardines, mackerel) to at least twice weekly.

References — Chapter Fifteen

Greenblatt, J.M. & Gottlieb, B. (2017). Finally Focused: The Breakthrough Natural Treatment Plan for ADHD. New York: Harmony Books.

Konofal, E. et al. (2004). 'Iron deficiency in children with ADHD.' Archives of Pediatrics and Adolescent Medicine, 158(12), 1113–1115.

Wan, L. et al. (2022). 'Association between MTHFR (677C>T and 1298A>C) polymorphisms and psychiatric disorder: a meta-analysis.' *PLOS ONE*, 17(7), e0271170.

Gokcen, C. et al. (2018). 'A contribution of methylenetetrahydrofolate reductase (MTHFR) gene polymorphisms in children with attention deficit hyperactivity disorder.' *Current Pediatric Research*, 22(4), 277–284.

Bilici, M. et al. (2004). 'Double-blind, placebo-controlled study of zinc sulfate in the treatment of ADHD.' Progress in Neuro-Psychopharmacology and Biological Psychiatry, 28(1), 181–190.

Akhondzadeh, S. et al. (2004). 'Zinc sulfate as an adjunct to methylphenidate for the treatment of ADHD in children: a double blind and randomized trial.' BMC Psychiatry, 4, 9.

Mohammadpour, N. et al. (2018). 'Effect of vitamin D supplementation as adjunctive therapy to methylphenidate on ADHD symptoms.' Nutritional Neuroscience, 21(3), 202–209.

Walsh, W.J. (2012). Nutrient Power: Heal Your Biochemistry and Heal Your Brain. New York: Skyhorse Publishing.

McCann, D. et al. (2007). 'Food additives and hyperactive behaviour in 3-year-old and 8/9-year-old children in the community.' The Lancet, 370(9598), 1560–1567.

Schrauzer, G.N. & Shrestha, K.P. (1990). 'Lithium in drinking water and the incidences of crimes, suicides, and arrests related to drug addictions.' Biological Trace Element Research, 25(2), 105–113.

Rucklidge, J.J. & Kaplan, B.J. (2014). 'Broad-spectrum micronutrient treatment for attention-deficit/hyperactivity disorder.' Expert Review of Neurotherapeutics, 14(3), 345–349.

Chapter Sixteen

The Second Brain and the First Problem

Gut health, the microbiome, and the gut-brain axis in ADHD

> ***DANIEL — Age 42:*** *Daniel has had IBS for twenty years. He has been told it is stress-related, which is certainly not wrong, but is also not the complete explanation. What nobody has mentioned is that the gut and the brain are in constant conversation — and that the gut, in this relationship, does most of the talking. Nobody has mentioned that the lining of his intestine is, in a very real sense, a second nervous system; that the state of his microbiome — shaped by a decade of processed food and more antibiotic courses than he can remember — has been quietly influencing his brain chemistry in ways that no amount of adjusting his prescription can fully compensate for. The psychiatrist trying to correct Daniel's neurotransmitter balance from the top down has, without knowing it, been working against a gut that has been undermining that effort from the bottom up. Daniel has been treated for a brain problem that begins, in significant part, considerably further south.*

The gut and the brain are in constant communication. This is not a metaphor. It is anatomy.

The vagus nerve — the longest cranial nerve in the body, running from the brainstem to the abdomen — carries signals in both directions, but approximately 80–90% of its fibres carry information from gut to brain rather than brain to gut. The enteric nervous system — the network of 100–500 million neurons embedded in the gastrointestinal tract — is sufficiently complex and autonomous that it is often called 'the second brain.' The gut microbiome — the 38 trillion microorganisms residing in the gastrointestinal tract — produces neurotransmitters (including 95% of the body's serotonin and approximately 50% of its dopamine precursors), modulates immune function, regulates intestinal permeability, and produces short-chain fatty acids that directly influence brain function. This is not an emerging fringe theory. It is mainstream neuroscience that is only now beginning to influence clinical practice.

In ADHD, the gut-brain axis matters in ways that are beginning to be documented with increasing specificity.

The Microbiome in ADHD — What the Evidence Shows

Multiple studies have found differences in gut microbiome composition between children and adults with ADHD and neurotypical controls. A 2017 pilot study by Aarts et al. identified specific microbial patterns associated with ADHD — particularly reduced diversity and altered ratios of key bacterial families. Subsequent research has found that ADHD is associated with reduced levels of Bifidobacterium and Lactobacillus species — bacteria that are significant producers of GABA and supporters of serotonin synthesis — and elevated levels of certain Clostridium species associated with increased intestinal permeability.

Intestinal permeability — sometimes called 'leaky gut' — refers to a condition in which the tight junctions between intestinal epithelial cells become compromised, allowing bacterial products, undigested food proteins, and inflammatory molecules to cross the gut lining into systemic circulation. These substances trigger immune activation, increase systemic inflammation, and compromise the blood-brain barrier — producing neuroinflammation that directly impairs prefrontal function and dopaminergic signalling. In a brain already neurochemically vulnerable, this inflammatory load is clinically significant.

The relationship appears bidirectional: ADHD-associated lifestyle patterns — irregular eating, poor sleep, high stress, antibiotic use — disrupt the microbiome, and a disrupted microbiome worsens the neurological environment, which worsens ADHD symptoms, which further disrupts lifestyle patterns. Breaking this cycle requires targeting the microbiome directly rather than waiting for downstream pharmacological corrections to work.

The Serotonin Connection — Why the Gut Matters for Mood

The fact that approximately 95% of the body's serotonin is produced in the gut — specifically in enterochromaffin cells of the intestinal lining, under the influence of the microbiome — has profound implications for ADHD management. Serotonin cannot cross the blood-brain barrier in its peripheral form; what the gut produces does not directly become brain serotonin. But gut serotonin is critical for gut motility, vagal nerve signalling, and the regulation of the gut-brain dialogue that shapes mood and cognition.

More directly: the microbiome influences the production of tryptophan — the amino acid precursor to serotonin — from dietary protein, and determines how much of that tryptophan is available for serotonin synthesis versus being metabolised along the kynurenine pathway (which produces inflammatory compounds including quinolinic acid, a glutamate receptor agonist with neurotoxic properties). A dysbiotic microbiome shifts tryptophan metabolism toward the kynurenine pathway, simultaneously reducing serotonin precursor availability and increasing neuroinflammatory load. For ADHD subtypes where serotonin is a primary target — Overfocused, Limbic, Ring of Fire — this is a clinically important mechanism that gut health intervention directly addresses.

Practical Gut Health — What to Do

The evidence base for microbiome intervention in ADHD specifically is still developing, but the foundational principles of gut health optimisation are well-established and broadly relevant to brain health across all ADHD subtypes.

Diet is the most powerful modulator of microbiome composition available. A diet high in diverse plant fibre — the prebiotic substrate that feeds beneficial bacteria — consistently increases microbiome diversity, which is the single most robustly associated feature of a healthy microbiome. The recommendation is straightforward in principle and challenging in the context of ADHD, where food selectivity, irregular eating patterns, and the dopaminergic pull toward high-sugar, low-fibre foods actively work against gut health: aim for 30 or more different plant species per week, including vegetables, fruits, legumes, whole grains, nuts, and seeds. Every additional species of plant food adds nutritional diversity that translates to microbial diversity.

Fermented foods — live-culture yoghurt, kefir, sauerkraut, kimchi, miso, kombucha — directly introduce beneficial bacteria and have been associated with improved microbiome diversity and reduced inflammatory markers in controlled studies. Introducing these foods gradually prevents the initial gastrointestinal discomfort that sometimes accompanies rapid microbiome changes.

Probiotic supplementation provides a more targeted approach. For ADHD, strains with specific evidence for ADHD-relevant outcomes include: Lactobacillus rhamnosus GG (which reduces anxiety-like behaviour in animal models through vagal GABA pathways), Bifidobacterium longum (which reduces cortisol response to stress and has demonstrated anxiolytic effects in human studies), and Lactobacillus acidophilus (which supports serotonin synthesis and intestinal barrier integrity). A comprehensive multi-strain probiotic containing at least 10 billion colony-forming units (CFU) is a reasonable starting point for most adults.

Avoiding microbiome disruptors is as important as introducing microbiome supports. Unnecessary antibiotic courses — particularly broad-spectrum antibiotics — produce profound and sometimes long-lasting microbiome disruption. Non-steroidal anti-inflammatory drugs (NSAIDs, including ibuprofen), taken regularly, impair intestinal barrier function. Artificial sweeteners — particularly saccharin, sucralose, and aspartame — alter microbiome composition in ways that increase glucose intolerance and, in some studies, increase inflammatory tone. Chronic stress — which is both a common feature and consequence of ADHD — elevates cortisol and reduces microbiome diversity through effects on intestinal motility and barrier function.

Omega-3 Fatty Acids and Gut-Brain Communication

Omega-3 fatty acids — discussed further in the supplementation chapter — have specific relevance to gut health that is often overlooked. EPA and DHA are incorporated into the cell membranes of intestinal epithelial cells, improving barrier function and reducing permeability. They modulate the production of short-chain fatty acids by the microbiome, increasing butyrate production — the primary fuel of colonocytes and a potent regulator of neuroinflammation. And they shift the eicosanoid balance away from the inflammatory prostaglandins produced by omega-6-dominated membranes toward anti-inflammatory resolvins and protectins.

The typical modern diet — high in omega-6 fatty acids from seed oils and processed foods, low in omega-3 from fatty fish and grass-fed animal products — produces a systemic inflammatory state that is both a consequence of poor gut health and a driver of it. The omega-6 to omega-3 ratio in the ancestral human diet is estimated to have been approximately 1:1 to 4:1; the modern Western diet commonly produces ratios of 15:1 to 20:1, a degree of imbalance that drives the chronic low-grade inflammation implicated in neuroinflammatory conditions including the Ring of Fire ADHD profile. Correcting this ratio through dietary modification and supplementation is one of the most broadly beneficial nutritional interventions for both gut and brain health.

For those who consume animal products, fatty fish — salmon, sardines, mackerel, anchovies, and herring — remain the most bioavailable and concentrated sources of the long-chain omega-3s EPA and DHA that the brain and gut directly utilise. Grass-fed butter and ghee contain higher omega-3 concentrations than their grain-fed equivalents and provide butyrate — a short-chain fatty acid that directly nourishes the intestinal lining — but their absolute omega-3 content remains modest and insufficient as a primary source, particularly for individuals with significant inflammatory burden or neurological goals.

For vegetarians and vegans, the picture requires careful navigation. Plant-based omega-3 sources — flaxseed, chia seeds, hemp seeds, and walnuts — provide alpha-linolenic acid (ALA), which the body must convert to the longer-chain EPA and DHA that confer neurological and anti-inflammatory benefit. This conversion is, in most people, inefficient: estimates suggest that only 5–10% of dietary ALA is converted to EPA, and less than 0.5–1% to DHA. For individuals with MTHFR variants, chronic inflammation, or high omega-6 intake — all common in ADHD populations — this conversion rate is further reduced. ALA-rich plant foods are therefore valuable but insufficient as the sole omega-3 strategy for brain health. The most important solution for vegetarians and vegans is algal oil — the direct marine algae from which fish themselves derive their EPA and DHA. Algal oil provides long-chain EPA and DHA without the fish, is environmentally sustainable, and is now widely available in capsule form. It is the recommended primary omega-3 supplement for anyone not consuming fatty fish regularly.

For cooking oils, the choice matters considerably. Extra virgin olive oil — high in oleic acid (omega-9) and polyphenols with minimal omega-6 — is the most evidence-supported culinary oil for both cardiovascular and neurological health and is stable at moderate cooking temperatures. Avocado oil has a similar profile and is more stable at higher heat. Flaxseed oil and hemp oil provide ALA and can be used cold — in dressings and smoothies — but should never be heated as they oxidise rapidly. Seed oils high in omega-6 — sunflower, safflower, corn, soybean, canola, and rice bran — should be minimised or eliminated regardless of dietary preference, as they are the primary driver of the omega-6 excess that shifts the balance toward systemic inflammation. Coconut oil, while saturated, has a neutral omega-6 profile and is stable at high heat, making it a reasonable cooking option when olive or avocado oil is not appropriate for the dish.

✦ Action Plan — Chapter Sixteen

→ Count your plant species per week. Aim for 30 or more different plant foods — count every variety separately (red and green lettuce are two different species). Use a notes app to track.

→ Add one or two fermented foods to your daily diet. Live-culture yoghurt at breakfast, a tablespoon of sauerkraut at lunch, or kefir in a smoothie. Start small if you are not used to fermented foods.

→ Begin a multi-strain probiotic (at least 5 different strains, at least 10 billion CFU) for 12 weeks. Take at a different time from any antibiotic courses. If you need to take antibiotics, double the probiotic dose during and for 4 weeks after.

→ Request a comprehensive stool analysis from your integrative practitioner if you have significant GI symptoms, have taken multiple antibiotic courses, or have persistent mental health symptoms that are poorly responsive to standard treatment.

→ Reduce artificial sweeteners to zero if possible — replace with small amounts of stevia (which has a more benign microbiome profile) or simply reduce sweet taste overall.

→ Increase dietary fibre gradually — if ADHD-related food selectivity is limiting variety, introduce fibre through means that work for your palate: smoothies, soups, mixed dishes where vegetables are less prominent texturally.

References — Chapter Sixteen

Aarts, E. et al. (2017). 'Gut microbiome in ADHD and its relation to neural reward anticipation.' PLoS ONE, 12(9), e0183509.

Cryan, J.F. et al. (2019). 'The microbiota-gut-brain axis.' Physiological Reviews, 99(4), 1877–2013.

Dinan, T.G. & Cryan, J.F. (2017). 'The microbiome-gut-brain axis in health and disease.' Gastroenterology Clinics of North America, 46(1), 77–89.

Sonnenburg, J. & Sonnenburg, E. (2015). The Good Gut. New York: Penguin Press.

Mayer, E.A. (2016). The Mind-Gut Connection. New York: HarperCollins.

Forsythe, P. et al. (2010). 'Mood and gut feelings.' Brain, Behaviour and Immunity, 24(1), 9–16.

Silk, D.B. et al. (2009). 'Clinical trial: the effects of a trans-galactooligosaccharide prebiotic on faecal microbiota and symptoms in irritable bowel syndrome.' Alimentary Pharmacology and Therapeutics, 29(5), 508–518.

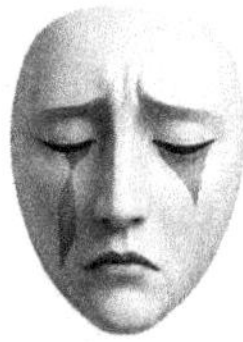

Chapter Seventeen

The Most Underrated Drug in Psychiatry

Sleep, the ADHD brain, revenge bedtime procrastination, and how to actually fix it

> ***PRIYA — Age 27:*** *She does not go to bed. This is not insomnia in the clinical sense — she is not lying awake unable to sleep. She simply does not go to bed. The evening is the only time in her day when nobody is demanding anything of her, when the calendar has no claims, when she can read what she wants or watch what she wants or think what she wants without it meaning she has failed at something. She knows she should sleep. She keeps choosing not to. It is 1:47 a.m. It has been 1:47 a.m. most nights for a decade. She is exhausted all day and suddenly alive at midnight. She has no idea why.*

Sleep is not a passive state. It is the period during which the brain performs its most critical maintenance operations: consolidating memories through hippocampal replay, clearing metabolic waste products (including amyloid-beta) via the glymphatic system, restoring prefrontal regulatory capacity depleted by the demands of the day, and resetting the dopaminergic reward machinery for the following morning's motivational landscape. A brain deprived of adequate sleep is not merely tired. It is neurobiologically impaired — in ways that are, in many cases, clinically indistinguishable from ADHD.

For the ADHD brain, sleep is both more important and harder to achieve than for the neurotypical brain. The reasons are multiple, interacting, and deeply rooted in the same neurobiological architecture that drives the attentional difficulties.

Why ADHD and Sleep Are Neurologically Intertwined

The relationship between ADHD and sleep runs deeper than 'hyperactive children don't settle down at night.' It is embedded in the same dopaminergic and circadian systems that drive the condition itself.

Circadian rhythm disruption is disproportionately common in ADHD: multiple studies have found delayed circadian phase in ADHD populations — a biological shift in the sleep-wake cycle toward later timing — that is distinct from mere behavioural delay. The CLOCK gene, which regulates circadian timing, has been identified as a candidate gene in ADHD susceptibility. The delay is not simply a preference for evenings; it is a biological shift in the timing of melatonin secretion, core body temperature nadir, and cortisol awakening response that can make both sleep onset and morning waking genuinely difficult, independently of any behavioural choices. Priya's 1:47 a.m. is not entirely a choice. Her circadian clock is running late, and has been since childhood.

Dopamine plays a critical role in circadian regulation — a largely underappreciated connection with direct clinical implications. The dopaminergic pathways involved in reward and motivation also regulate sleep-wake transitions, and the reduced dopaminergic tone characteristic of Classic and Inattentive ADHD is associated with weaker circadian signal strength — a less pronounced biological distinction between daytime alertness and nighttime sleep drive. This produces the characteristic ADHD sleep profile: difficulty initiating sleep at a conventional time, often delayed sleep onset by 1–3 hours, difficulty waking in the morning (which is not laziness but genuine biological misalignment), and a pattern of performing at one's best in the late evening when circadian phase finally aligns with waking function.

Sleep disorders are independently prevalent in ADHD: restless legs syndrome (RLS) affects approximately 25% of ADHD individuals compared to 5% of the general population. RLS involves uncomfortable sensations in the legs at rest, particularly in the evening, that compel movement — directly disrupting sleep initiation. The shared neurobiological basis (dopaminergic insufficiency in both RLS and ADHD) explains the co-occurrence. Sleep apnoea and upper airway resistance syndrome are also more prevalent in ADHD populations and produce fragmented, non-restorative sleep that compounds the pre-existing neurological vulnerabilities.

Revenge Bedtime Procrastination — The ADHD Phenomenon with a Name

The concept of revenge bedtime procrastination has entered popular vocabulary in recent years — the pattern of deliberately staying up late not because of insomnia but as a form of resistance to days that feel entirely spent under others' demands. The 'revenge' is reclaiming personal time from a schedule that otherwise allows none. The ADHD dimension of this is specific and important.

For individuals with ADHD, and particularly those in the inattentive and overfocused presentations, the daytime is frequently experienced as a sustained performance — maintaining the focus, the organisation, the social presentation, the executive function demands of work, school, and relationship — that leaves little genuine psychic space for self-directed activity. The evening, when those demands lift, is neurologically different: lower social expectation, lower performance pressure, and consequently reduced inhibition on the brain's own meandering, hyperfocusing, and freely associating tendencies. This combination of reduced external demand and increased internal freedom is genuinely restorative in a way that the day is not — and it happens to coincide with the period when the circadian-delayed ADHD brain is beginning to feel most awake.

The result is a pattern of late-night engagement — reading, watching, gaming, thinking, creating — followed by inadequate sleep, followed by impaired morning functioning, followed by a depleted day that makes the evening's privacy even more precious and the following night's procrastination even more likely. This cycle is not a character failing. It is a rational response to a genuinely inadequate life structure, embedded in a neurobiological tendency toward delayed phase and an understandable resistance to days that feel overdrawn from the start.

Addressing revenge bedtime procrastination requires addressing the conditions that make it rewarding — not simply adding a bedtime alarm. If the daytime provides no genuine restorative activities, no sense of personal autonomy, no spaces for the ADHD brain's natural tendencies to operate without penalty, the evening will continue to be defended. Building protected daytime spaces — periods of genuinely self-directed activity, creative engagement, or solitary recovery — reduces the pressure on the evening and makes earlier sleep a smaller sacrifice.

Sleep Hygiene — What Actually Works

'Sleep hygiene' has become something of a clinical cliché — a list of commonsense recommendations that patients receive and usually do not implement, partly because of the difficulty with routine that characterises ADHD and partly because the recommendations are delivered without acknowledgement of the specific barriers that ADHD creates. A sleep hygiene protocol for an ADHD brain needs to be designed for an ADHD brain.

Light management is the single most evidence-based behavioural sleep intervention. The circadian clock is primarily set by light — specifically blue-wavelength light detected by intrinsically photosensitive retinal ganglion cells that project directly to the suprachiasmatic nucleus (the brain's master clock). Bright blue light exposure in the evening delays melatonin secretion and pushes the circadian clock later — precisely the wrong direction for the already-delayed ADHD circadian profile. Reducing blue light exposure after 8 p.m. (screens, overhead LED lighting), using blue-blocking glasses or red-shifted evening lighting, and ensuring bright natural light exposure in the first thirty minutes of morning waking are the most physiologically specific behavioural interventions available. The morning light exposure is as important as the evening blue-light reduction: it advances the circadian clock and strengthens the signal strength that weakly circadian ADHD brains need. The simplest and most underrated implementation strategy for morning light exposure requires no alarm, no lamp purchase, and no additional time: sleep with the blinds or curtains open. Natural light entering the room at dawn triggers the cortisol awakening response and begins advancing the circadian clock before the eyes are even fully open — making the biological work of waking up a passive process rather than a daily battle against a darkened room and a body that has received no signal that morning has arrived.

Temperature regulation: core body temperature must fall approximately 1–2°C for sleep to initiate and maintain. A cool bedroom (approximately 16–19°C) supports this fall. A warm bath or shower 60–90 minutes before bedtime paradoxically accelerates the temperature drop by dilating peripheral blood vessels and dissipating heat — a technique with specific evidence for sleep onset latency reduction.

Stimulus control — using the bed only for sleep and (where relevant) sex, not for screens, reading, or working — remains one of the most evidence-based behavioural recommendations. For ADHD, where work frequently migrates to the bedroom because of time blindness and last-minute urgency, this boundary is particularly important and particularly difficult to maintain. External structure helps: a physically separate charging station for devices outside the bedroom removes the option.

Consistent wake time — maintained even after poor sleep — is the most powerful circadian anchor available. Variable wake time, which is extremely common in ADHD (sleeping in on weekends to recover from the week's deficit), fragments the circadian signal and perpetuates the delayed phase. One fixed wake time, maintained seven days a week, is more effective than any sleep medication for circadian phase alignment. It is also, for most people with ADHD, the most difficult sleep recommendation to implement. Which is why the following section matters.

Melatonin — Useful, Misunderstood, and Usually Misused

Melatonin is the hormone that signals darkness to the body — secreted by the pineal gland in response to the absence of light, it does not cause sleep but communicates the timing of night and prepares the body's systems for sleep. It is the most commonly used sleep supplement across the world and, in ADHD specifically, has the most extensive evidence base of any sleep intervention.

The good news: melatonin is effective for ADHD. A systematic review and meta-analysis found that melatonin significantly reduces sleep onset latency in children with ADHD — helping them fall asleep earlier — with a good safety profile and minimal side effects at appropriate doses (Cortese et al., 2020). For circadian delay specifically, melatonin taken 30–90 minutes before the desired sleep time (not at the current sleep time) acts as a circadian signal rather than a sedative, advancing the phase of melatonin secretion and progressively shifting the sleep window earlier. This is the correct use of melatonin: a chronobiotic signal, not a sleeping pill.

The not-so-good news: melatonin is almost universally misused in clinical and consumer practice. Most people take it too late (at bedtime, rather than 60–90 minutes before desired sleep onset), at too high a dose (many commercial preparations contain 5–10 mg, whereas the physiologically active dose is 0.1–0.5 mg — taking 10 mg of melatonin is like taking 40 times the effective dose and expecting better results), and without addressing the underlying circadian disruption that requires a sustained chronobiotic approach rather than a nightly pill.

The limitations of melatonin are equally important to communicate: it does not address sleep maintenance difficulties (waking during the night), it does not improve sleep architecture (the distribution of light, deep, and REM sleep), and it does not compensate for inadequate sleep duration. For sleep apnoea, restless legs, or anxiety-driven insomnia, melatonin addresses none of the underlying pathology and is correspondingly ineffective.

Sleep Medications — A Nuanced View

Prescription sleep medications — benzodiazepines (temazepam, diazepam), non-benzodiazepine 'Z-drugs' (zopiclone, zolpidem), and antihistamines (diphenhydramine) — are widely prescribed for sleep difficulties in ADHD and share a common limitation: they produce sedation rather than sleep. The neurological architecture of pharmacologically sedated sleep is different from the architecture of natural sleep — it suppresses slow-wave sleep and REM disproportionately, compromising the memory consolidation and emotional processing functions that make sleep neurologically restorative. In the short term, these medications reduce the subjective distress of lying awake. In the longer term, they impair the quality of the sleep they produce and risk dependence.

For ADHD specifically, sedating medications carry an additional concern: they do not address the underlying circadian delay or the neurobiological hyperarousal that drives sleep initiation difficulty in many subtypes (particularly Anxious, Ring of Fire, and Overfocused). They are also contraindicated in sleep apnoea, which co-occurs with ADHD at elevated rates. In the opinion of the authors, sleep medications should be last-resort short-term interventions rather than maintenance treatments — and any decision to prescribe them should be accompanied by evaluation for sleep apnoea and restless legs, and by active implementation of the behavioural and chronobiotic approaches described above.

There are exceptions: low-dose quetiapine, used as a sleep aid, has a somewhat different profile and may be appropriate in specific presentations where anxiety and rumination are primary sleep disruptors. Low-dose doxepin has specific evidence for sleep maintenance insomnia. A more recent pharmacological development worth noting is the emergence of orexin receptor antagonists — suvorexant (Belsomra) and lemborexant (Dayvigo) — as a genuinely different approach to sleep pharmacology in ADHD. Unlike traditional sedatives, which broadly suppress CNS activity, orexin antagonists work by blocking the neuropeptide responsible for maintaining wakefulness — allowing the brain's own sleep mechanisms to operate rather than forcing sedation. This produces sleep that more closely resembles natural sleep in its architecture, without the rebound insomnia, dependence risk, or next-day cognitive impairment associated with benzodiazepines and Z-drugs. For individuals with ADHD whose insomnia is driven by hyperarousal and an inability to disengage the wakefulness system — particularly Anxious and Ring of Fire subtypes — this mechanism is neurobiologically well-suited, and their profile makes them a more rational option for longer-term management than conventional sleep medications. The evidence base in ADHD-specific insomnia remains limited, and their interaction with stimulant medications warrants clinical monitoring. An important caution: orexin antagonists carry a documented risk of parasomnias — including sleep paralysis, hypnagogic hallucinations, and complex sleep behaviours such as sleepwalking — which, while uncommon, are more likely in individuals already vulnerable to sleep architecture disruption, as many with ADHD are. These are prescription medications requiring specialist assessment, not first-line interventions.

For individuals with Classic, Ring of Fire, or Anxious ADHD — where hyperarousal and an overactive sympathetic nervous system are primary drivers of sleep difficulty — clonidine is one of the most clinically useful and underutilised sleep interventions available. Its alpha-2 adrenergic agonism reduces noradrenergic outflow, quietens sympathetic arousal, and produces a physiological calm well-suited to the overactivated ADHD nervous system at night. At low doses — typically 0.05–0.1 mg taken 30–60 minutes before bed — it reliably reduces sleep onset latency, improves sleep continuity, and reduces nocturnal restlessness. Its sedating effect, a liability in daytime dosing, becomes an asset at bedtime. Clonidine has decades of evidence in paediatric ADHD populations specifically, is inexpensive, and can be effective in adults as well at similar doses. The primary cautions are rebound hypertension and insomnia on abrupt discontinuation — always taper — and additive hypotensive effects when combined with other antihypertensive agents.

Magnesium glycinate taken at bedtime — discussed in the supplementation chapter — has a well-established and physiologically logical role in sleep: magnesium modulates GABA receptors (reducing neuronal excitability and supporting sleep onset), regulates melatonin production, and reduces the muscle tension and restless legs symptoms that disturb sleep in many ADHD individuals. At doses of 200–400 mg elemental magnesium (as glycinate, for superior absorption and GI tolerance), taken 30–60 minutes before bed, it is among the most evidence-informed and safest sleep interventions available.

✦ Action Plan — Chapter Seventeen

→ Set one fixed wake time and maintain it seven days a week for 4 weeks. This is the most powerful single circadian intervention. It will be difficult for the first 1–2 weeks. Persist.

→ Get bright light exposure within 30 minutes of waking — go outside, or use a 10,000 lux light therapy lamp for 20–30 minutes at breakfast. This is the morning anchor for the circadian clock.

→ Put on blue-blocking glasses at 8 p.m. or switch all screens to night mode and switch overhead lights to red-shifted warm bulbs. Blue light after sunset delays melatonin secretion by up to 3 hours.

→ If using melatonin, switch to 0.3–0.5 mg (not 5–10 mg) taken 90 minutes before your desired sleep time, not your current sleep time. This is chronobiotic use, not sedative use.

→ Take magnesium glycinate 200–400 mg elemental magnesium 30–60 minutes before bed. If you have restless legs in the evenings, this is especially relevant.

→ Create a transition buffer: 30 minutes to an hour before bed, stop screens, reduce light, and do one low-stimulus activity (reading physical books, gentle stretching, a warm bath). Your brain needs a physiological ramp-down that it will not initiate spontaneously.

→ Identify your personal revenge bedtime procrastination pattern and schedule 30–45 minutes of protected, guilt-free self-directed time in the afternoon or early evening — before the evening begins. This reduces the pressure on late-night hours.

References — Chapter Seventeen

Cortese, S. et al. (2020). 'Sleep in ADHD: a systematic review and framework for future research.' Sleep Medicine Reviews, 52, 101330.

Van der Heijden, K.B. et al. (2007). 'Effect of melatonin on sleep, behavior, and cognition in ADHD and chronic sleep-onset insomnia.' Journal of the American Academy of Child & Adolescent Psychiatry, 46(2), 233–241.

Hvolby, A. (2015). 'Associations of sleep disturbance with ADHD.' ADHD Attention Deficit and Hyperactivity Disorders, 7(1), 1–18.

Walker, M. (2017). Why We Sleep. New York: Scribner.

Phillips, A.J.K. et al. (2017). 'Irregular sleep/wake patterns are associated with poorer academic performance and delayed circadian and sleep/wake timing.' Scientific Reports, 7, 3216.

Eckerberg, B. et al. (2012). 'Melatonin treatment effects on adolescent students' sleep timing and sleepiness in a placebo-controlled crossover study.' Chronobiology International, 29(9), 1239–1248.

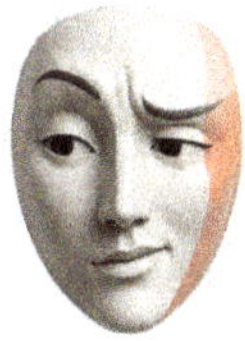

Chapter Eighteen

Movement, Molecules, and the Subtype-Specific Supplement Plan

Exercise as medicine, digital detox, and what your neurotype actually needs

> ***LIAM — Age 25:*** *The one thing that has consistently worked, throughout his life, without a prescription, without side effects, without a waiting list: skateboarding. Not because skateboarding is particularly virtuous — it has cost him three fractured wrists and one suspended sentence — but because the physical intensity, the proprioceptive feedback, the moment-by-moment demand for total concentration, and the dopaminergic payoff of successfully landing a trick produce exactly the neurological state that nothing else in his day generates. He just didn't know it had a mechanism.*

Exercise — The Intervention That Nobody Prescribes

If exercise came in a pill, it would be the most prescribed medication in psychiatry. The evidence for its effects on ADHD is, for the relevant outcomes, comparable to stimulant medication — and for some outcomes, superior to it. Unlike stimulant medication, exercise produces durable neurological changes rather than temporary symptom suppression. Unlike stimulant medication, it improves cardiovascular health, metabolic function, and sleep architecture simultaneously. Unlike stimulant medication, it has no abuse potential, no tolerance development, and no prescription requirement.

The neurological mechanism of exercise's effects on ADHD is well-documented. A single bout of moderate-to-vigorous aerobic exercise increases prefrontal dopamine and noradrenaline availability for 60–90 minutes following the session — the temporal window of enhanced cognitive function that teachers have known about empirically (putting PE before maths) for decades before the mechanism was identified. Over time, regular aerobic exercise increases BDNF (brain-derived neurotrophic factor) expression in the prefrontal cortex and hippocampus, supporting the neuroplasticity that underpins lasting improvement in executive function. It reduces elevated basal cortisol — the chronic stress response that impairs prefrontal function — and improves HRV, the autonomic regulation metric that is reduced in ADHD and Anxious ADHD specifically.

The dose-response relationship is important for practice: the effects on ADHD-relevant outcomes are most pronounced with moderate-to-vigorous intensity exercise (not leisurely walking), sustained for at least 20–30 minutes, aerobic in nature (running, cycling, swimming, rowing, team sports), and ideally performed in the morning to maximise the benefit during the school or working day. Exercise timing relative to cognitively demanding tasks appears to matter: performing 20–30 minutes of vigorous aerobic activity immediately before sustained cognitive work produces the largest acute attentional benefit. For children with ADHD, this has obvious implications for school scheduling.

High-intensity interval training (HIIT) produces the largest acute dopaminergic response per unit of time and may be particularly useful for the time-pressed adult with ADHD who cannot sustain thirty continuous minutes of lower-intensity effort. Mind-body exercises — martial arts, gymnastics, yoga, dance — add proprioceptive and attentional demands that appear to augment the neurological benefit beyond that of equivalent aerobic intensity alone. For Classic and Anxious ADHD specifically, activities with external structure and clear performance feedback (team sports, competitive athletics) harness the motivational architecture of these subtypes — external accountability and concrete outcome metrics — in ways that unstructured gym sessions typically cannot.

Digital Detox — The Environment That Makes Everything Worse

The ADHD brain and the attention economy are locked in a relationship that is deeply, specifically hostile to everything this book has been advocating. Every feature of the modern digital environment — infinite scroll, variable reward notifications, algorithmically curated novelty, frictionless switching between stimuli — is engineered to exploit precisely the neurological vulnerabilities that characterise ADHD: impaired inhibitory control, novelty-seeking, Salience Network overresponsiveness to immediate stimulation, and susceptibility to dopaminergic hijacking.

Johann Hari's *Stolen Focus* (2022) makes the compelling case that what looks like an epidemic of individual attentional failure is, in significant part, a designed outcome — that the attention economy has been deliberately engineered to overwhelm the very cognitive systems that regulate focus, and that the ADHD brain, already operating with reduced inhibitory control and heightened novelty-seeking, is not merely susceptible to this environment but is, in a very real sense, its most profitable customer. The book is recommended reading for anyone who has wondered why their strategies for managing distraction keep failing despite genuine effort — and for any clinician who has advised a patient to simply put their phone down, without fully reckoning with what that phone has been designed to prevent them from doing.

What we are contending with is not merely excessive screen time. It is a progressive degradation of the attentional capacity that ADHD brains have in limited supply. Research has demonstrated that heavy social media use is associated with increased ADHD symptoms in non-ADHD individuals — the attentional demands of the digital environment are sufficient to produce ADHD-like symptoms in neurotypical brains. For ADHD brains, the effect is amplified: the same features that make social media compulsively engaging (variable reward, novelty, social validation loops) also make sustained, effortful, non-digital work progressively less tolerable by comparison.

Digital detox does not mean abandoning technology. It means restructuring its use in ways that reduce its capacity to degrade attentional baseline. Specific evidence-informed strategies include: notification management (turning off all non-essential notifications — the average smartphone user receives 65–80 notifications per day, each representing an attentional interruption that takes 23 minutes to fully recover from in terms of focused work); app usage limits set externally and made difficult to override in the moment; grayscale screen mode (which reduces the visual salience of app icons and slows compulsive checking); and structured technology-free periods (at minimum: no screens for 60 minutes after waking and 60 minutes before sleep).

The specific impact of gaming on ADHD merits separate acknowledgement. Gaming is highly rewarding for ADHD brains — the structure of rewards, the clear objectives, the immediate feedback, and the social connection all speak directly to the motivational architecture of the dopamine-seeking ADHD neurotype. In moderation, gaming can be a genuine source of engagement, social connection, and even cognitive training. In excess — particularly in the context of poor sleep, inadequate exercise, and suboptimal academic or occupational functioning — it becomes the default activity that ADHD brains migrate toward at the expense of everything else. The clinical position is not condemnation but calibration: if gaming is occurring at the expense of sleep, relationships, or functional responsibilities, it requires the same structural management as any other addictive behaviour.

Neurofeedback — Mindfulness on Steroids

Mindfulness meditation has a well-documented evidence base for anxiety, depression, and stress reduction, and a growing evidence base for ADHD specifically: mindfulness training increases prefrontal grey matter density, reduces default mode network overactivity during tasks, and improves attention regulation in controlled trials (Zylowska et al., 2008; Mitchell et al., 2013). In an ideal world, a daily 20–30 minute mindfulness practice would be a standard recommendation for every ADHD subtype.

In the real world, mindfulness meditation is extraordinarily difficult for many people with ADHD. The practice requires the practitioner to direct and sustain attention voluntarily — precisely the capacity that is most neurologically limited in ADHD. 'Notice when your attention wanders and gently return it to the breath' is, for many ADHD brains, an instruction to notice their attention wandering and then struggle to return it, repeatedly, while experiencing escalating frustration at the difficulty of what should be simple. Many people with ADHD who have attempted meditation report that it feels like 'failing at relaxing' — a particularly unhelpful psychological experience for a population with already heightened sensitivity to failure and self-criticism.

This is where neurofeedback becomes relevant in a way that goes beyond its use as an ADHD treatment protocol. Neurofeedback is, in its fundamental mechanism, assisted mindfulness: real-time feedback from the brain's own electrical signals allows the individual to become aware of their internal states — the shift from theta-dominant unfocused mind-wandering to beta-dominant engaged attention, the reduction of high-beta anxious overactivation, the deepening of alpha-rhythm relaxed awareness — and to learn to modulate those states through a training process that leverages the brain's neuroplastic capacity.

Long-term practitioners of deep meditation — Tibetan Buddhist monks, experienced Vipassana meditators — show brain electrical patterns characterised by increased gamma-band synchrony, elevated frontal alpha coherence, and rapid transitions between attentional states that are strikingly similar to the targets of advanced neurofeedback training. The subjective experience of sustained, effortless presence — the 'flow state' that meditation seeks and that ADHD brains access primarily through hyperfocus — appears to correspond to specific EEG patterns that neurofeedback can train directly.

For individuals with ADHD who have found conventional meditation inaccessible, neurofeedback offers a technology-assisted entry point to states of regulated attention that might otherwise take years of dedicated practice to access. The feedback provides what the ADHD brain needs: immediate, objective, external information about an internal state, replacing the abstract instruction to 'be mindful' with a concrete, measurable training target. Patients consistently report that effective neurofeedback produces subjective experiences of calm, clarity, and mental spaciousness that they previously associated only with their best days — and that with repeated training, the ability to access those states voluntarily becomes increasingly available outside the neurofeedback session itself.

Subtype-Specific Supplement Protocols

The foundational supplements described in Chapter Fifteen — omega-3 fatty acids, magnesium, zinc, vitamin D — apply across all ADHD subtypes and should be established before introducing subtype-specific additions. The following section is only intended as a guide. Many supplements have interactions with medications and it is vital to seek the opinion of a qualified practitioner before starting subtype-specific supplements.

Foundational — All Subtypes

Omega-3 fatty acids: EPA-dominant formula (minimum 1g EPA daily, ideally 2–3g for brain health and anti-inflammatory effects). Fish oil, algal oil for vegetarians/vegans. Quality matters: look for third-party testing for mercury and PCBs.

Magnesium glycinate: 200–400 mg elemental magnesium daily, ideally split morning and bedtime.

Zinc glycinate or picolinate: 15–25 mg daily, taken with food.

Vitamin D3 with K2: 2000–5000 IU D3 with 100–200 μg MK-7 K2, taken with a fat-containing meal.

Classic ADHD — Dopaminergic Support

L-Tyrosine: 500–2000 mg in the morning on an empty stomach. Tyrosine is the direct amino acid precursor to dopamine and noradrenaline; supplementation supports the dopamine synthesis pathway that is the primary neurochemical target of this subtype. Best used on stimulant-free days, medication holidays, or as an adjunct to reduce stimulant dose.

Rhodiola rosea: 200–400 mg of standardised extract (3% rosavins, 1% salidroside) in the morning. An adaptogenic herb with documented effects on dopaminergic signalling, fatigue resistance, and stress cortisol reduction — particularly relevant for the executive fatigue that characterises Classic ADHD by afternoon.

Oligomeric proanthocyanidins (OPCs) from grape seed or pine bark extract: 100–200 mg daily. Multiple randomised trials have found significant improvements in ADHD symptoms with maritime pine bark extract (Pycnogenol) — effect attributed to antioxidant protection of dopaminergic neurons and anti-inflammatory action.

Panax ginseng: 200–400 mg standardised extract daily. Has documented effects on dopaminergic activity and sustained attention in randomised trials in ADHD populations.

Inattentive ADHD — Alpha and Attention

L-Tyrosine: as above, with particular relevance to the dopaminergic contributions to the inattentive profile.

SAMe (S-adenosylmethionine): 400–800 mg daily in the morning, on an empty stomach. SAMe is a methyl donor involved in the synthesis of both dopamine and serotonin, and has demonstrated antidepressant and pro-attentional effects. Particularly relevant for inattentive presentations with low mood and low hedonic tone.

Acetyl-L-carnitine: 500–2000 mg daily. Has specific evidence in ADHD from two randomised trials, with particular benefit for the inattentive profile. Supports mitochondrial energy metabolism in neurons and modulates cholinergic function relevant to attention networks.

Overfocused ADHD — Serotonergic Flexibility

5-HTP (5-hydroxytryptophan): 50–100 mg, typically taken in the evening. The immediate precursor to serotonin; supports serotonin synthesis for the anterior cingulate circuits that drive perseveration in this subtype. Should not be combined with SSRIs or SNRIs without medical supervision.

Inositol: 12–18 g daily (best taken as a powder in water, divided across the day). Has the most evidence in OCD — the condition most closely related to the Overfocused profile — from multiple randomised trials. Modulates serotonin receptor sensitivity and inositol signalling cascade.

Saffron (Crocus sativus): 30 mg standardised extract (safranal and crocin) twice daily. Has demonstrated antidepressant and anti-obsessional effects in controlled trials, with a mechanism involving serotonin reuptake inhibition similar to SSRIs but without the side effect profile. Relevant across Overfocused, Limbic, and Ring of Fire profiles.

L-Theanine: 100–200 mg with morning coffee or tea. Promotes calm alertness by increasing alpha and GABA activity; specifically counteracts the rigid hyperalertness of the Overfocused profile.

Magnesium glycinate: higher end of the dosing range (400 mg elemental) for its glutamate-modulating effects at the ACC.

Temporal Lobe ADHD — Stability and GABA Support

GABA (gamma-aminobutyric acid): 250–750 mg in the evening. While exogenous GABA has variable CNS penetration, some individuals report benefit, and it is generally safe. Pharma GABA (produced by fermentation) may have superior CNS activity.

Magnesium glycinate: as above, with specific relevance to GABA receptor modulation and temporal lobe stabilisation.

L-Theanine: 200 mg evening dose, for alpha-promoting and GABA-supporting effects.

Pyridoxal-5-phosphate (P5P): 25–50 mg daily. The active form of B6, essential for GABA synthesis — important in Temporal Lobe profiles where GABA deficiency is a primary target. A note of caution: prolonged supplementation with vitamin B6 at high doses above 50 mg daily has been associated with peripheral neuropathy but is considerably lower with P5P. Nevertheless, B6 supplementation at any dose should not be open-ended and periodic review is essential.

Taurine: 500–1000 mg. An inhibitory neuromodulator with GABA-mimetic properties and specific evidence for reducing temporal lobe excitability.

Limbic ADHD — Mood and Motivation

EPA-rich omega-3: increase to 2–3g EPA daily; the evidence for EPA specifically as an antidepressant and mood stabiliser is stronger than for DHA.

5-HTP: 50–100 mg evening dose, supporting serotonin synthesis for the mood regulatory circuits.

Saffron extract: 30 mg twice daily — has demonstrated antidepressant effects comparable to fluoxetine in controlled trials, with relevance to the low-hedonic-tone of the Limbic profile.

SAMe: 400–800 mg daily, for combined dopaminergic and serotonergic support.

L-Tyrosine: morning dose for dopaminergic motivation support.

Zinc: at the higher end of dosing (25 mg) for its antidepressant properties.

Ring of Fire ADHD — Calming the Overheated Cortex

GABA and L-Theanine: as per Temporal Lobe protocol, with emphasis on the calming and alpha-promoting effects.

Magnesium glycinate: 400 mg elemental, for NMDA receptor blockade and glutamate excess reduction.

NAC (N-acetylcysteine): 600–1200 mg twice daily. Modulates glutamate release through the cystine-glutamate antiporter; has the most established evidence base for glutamate-excess conditions (trichotillomania, OCD, bipolar disorder). Relevant for Ring of Fire's glutamate excess neurochemistry.

Saffron: 30 mg twice daily, for its anti-inflammatory and serotonergic effects.

EPA omega-3: 2–3g daily for anti-inflammatory action. Avoid high-dose stimulating supplements (high-dose tyrosine, rhodiola, ginseng) that increase cortical arousal.

Anxious ADHD — Calming Without Sedating

L-Theanine: 200 mg, can be taken up to twice daily. The calm-alertness effect is specifically suited to Anxious ADHD — increases alpha and GABA without sedation, allowing the attentional components to function more effectively in a less anxious internal environment.

Magnesium glycinate: as above.

Ashwagandha (Withania somnifera): 300–600 mg of KSM-66 extract twice daily. Has the most robust evidence base of any adaptogen for anxiety reduction — multiple randomised trials demonstrate significant reduction in cortisol, generalised anxiety, and perceived stress without sedation or dependence.

Inositol: 12–18 g daily, for the anxiety-OCD dimension often present.

HRV biofeedback: not a supplement but the most evidence-based non-pharmacological intervention for Anxious ADHD's autonomic dysregulation — free apps (Cohérence, eSense) make the 6-breaths-per-minute resonant frequency breathing practice accessible without equipment.

✦ Action Plan — Chapter Eighteen

→ Begin with the foundational four — omega-3, magnesium glycinate, zinc, vitamin D — before adding subtype-specific supplements. Establish the foundation for 4 weeks, then layer in subtype-specific additions.

→ Schedule 20–30 minutes of aerobic exercise on at least 5 days per week. For best cognitive results, perform it in the morning, before your most demanding cognitive work. Walking at moderate pace does not count — it needs to elevate your heart rate.

→ If you find meditation difficult, try a single 20-minute neurofeedback-informed breathing practice: breathe at 6 breaths per minute (5 seconds in, 5 seconds out) while noticing when your attention drifts and gently returning it. This is the physiological substrate of mindfulness with a built-in anchor.

→ Conduct a notification audit: turn off all social media, news, and non-essential app notifications. Leave only calls, calendar reminders, and messaging from your highest-priority contacts. Do this today.

→ Identify your subtype from Part Two and add the relevant 1–2 priority subtype supplements to your foundational four. Introduce one new supplement per week to track its individual effect.

→ If you use gaming as a primary coping mechanism, set a structural limit: a fixed end time (not a duration limit, which requires ongoing executive function to monitor) enforced by an external app or device timer that requires effort to override.

References — Chapter Eighteen

Ratey, J.J. & Hagerman, E. (2008). Spark: The Revolutionary New Science of Exercise and the Brain. New York: Little, Brown.

Pontifex, M.B. et al. (2013). 'Exercise improves behavioral, neurocognitive, and scholastic performance in children with ADHD.' Journal of Pediatrics, 162(3), 543–551.

Hari, J. (2022). *Stolen Focus: Why You Can't Pay Attention — and How to Think Deeply Again*. London: Bloomsbury Publishing.

Zylowska, L. et al. (2008). 'Mindfulness meditation training in adults and adolescents with ADHD.' Journal of Attention Disorders, 11(6), 737–746.

Mitchell, J.T. et al. (2013). 'A pilot trial of mindfulness meditation training for ADHD in adulthood: impact on core symptoms, executive functioning, and emotion dysregulation.' Journal of Attention Disorders, 19(11), 1105–1120.

Trebatická, J. et al. (2006). 'Treatment of ADHD with French maritime pine bark extract Pycnogenol.' European Child & Adolescent Psychiatry, 15(6), 329–335.

Ghanizadeh, A. et al. (2013). 'Zinc supplementation for ADHD: a randomized double-blind placebo controlled trial.' Nutritional Neuroscience, 16(4), 173–178.

Akhondzadeh, S. et al. (2010). 'Saffron in the treatment of children with ADHD: a randomized, double-blind trial.' Progress in Neuro-Psychopharmacology and Biological Psychiatry, 34(1), 76–80.

Chandrasekhar, K. et al. (2012). 'A prospective, randomized double-blind, placebo-controlled study of safety and efficacy of a high-concentration full-spectrum extract of ashwagandha root.' Indian Journal of Psychological Medicine, 34(3), 255–262.

Shanahan, L. et al. (2019). 'Emotional suppression and screen time in adolescents.' JAMA Pediatrics, 173(5), 446–452.

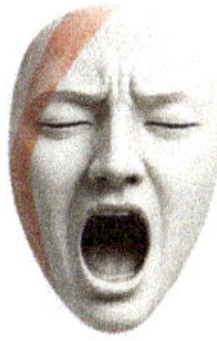

Chapter Nineteen

Training the Brain That Was Never Trained

Neurofeedback — what it is, how it works, what the evidence shows, and what to expect

> ***ZARA — Age 28, Three Months into Neurofeedback:*** *She was told at the outset to expect the first few sessions to feel strange, possibly frustrating, occasionally to temporarily worsen symptoms as the brain began to reorganise. The practitioner was accurate on all three counts. By session eight, something began to shift — not dramatically, not all at once, but a quality of quiet she had not previously experienced without sedation. By session twenty, she described it to her mother as: 'It feels like someone turned the volume down on everything. I can still hear it. I just don't have to fight it anymore.'*

Neurofeedback is one of those interventions that sounds, when described simply, almost too good to be true: you sit in a comfortable chair, wear some sensors on your scalp, watch a screen or listen to audio, and your brain learns to regulate itself. No drugs. No side effects. No injections. No radiation. And, if done correctly by a qualified practitioner using QEEG-guided protocols, lasting neurophysiological change — the kind that continues after the training stops, unlike the symptom suppression that ends when the medication does.

It sounds too good to be true partly because it is sold badly: marketed with excessive claims, offered by under-qualified practitioners using generic protocols, and applied to everyone with an ADHD diagnosis regardless of their QEEG profile, their subtype, or the appropriateness of the specific protocol for their brain. In those hands, neurofeedback underperforms its potential and gives sceptics legitimate ammunition.

Done well — by a BCIA-accredited practitioner, guided by a QEEG, adapted to the individual's neurophysiological profile, monitored continuously and adjusted as the brain changes — neurofeedback is one of the most evidence-based, neurobiologically coherent, and clinically significant interventions available for ADHD. This chapter makes the case for it, honestly, with the evidence as its foundation.

What Neurofeedback Actually Is

Neurofeedback is a form of biofeedback in which the physiological signal being fed back to the individual is the brain's own electrical activity — specifically, the EEG recorded in real time from electrodes placed on the scalp. The fundamental principle is operant conditioning: when the brain produces electrical activity within a desired frequency range (the 'reward' band), the feedback system produces a positive signal — a visual reward on screen, an audio tone, a video that plays smoothly. When the brain's activity moves outside the desired range, the feedback stops or changes. Through thousands of repetitions across multiple sessions, the brain learns — not through conscious effort or insight, but through the same neuroplastic mechanisms that underlie all learning — to spend more time in the rewarded state and less time in the unrewarded one.

The feedback is immediate: the lag between the brain producing a pattern and the system signalling its presence is typically less than 100 milliseconds — well within the window that supports conditioning. The individual does not need to understand what is happening neurologically. They do not need to consciously try to produce the desired pattern. The brain's conditioning mechanisms operate below the level of conscious awareness, which is why neurofeedback works for young children who cannot engage with the cognitive demands of CBT, and for adults with ADHD who cannot sustain voluntary attentional effort long enough to benefit from mindfulness practice.

The training session itself is typically 30–45 minutes. The individual sits comfortably — sometimes watching a film that plays clearly when the brain is in the reward state and dims or pauses when it is not; sometimes playing a simple computer game that responds to their brain activity rather than their keystrokes; sometimes simply listening to music that shifts in volume or quality based on their EEG. The subjective experience for most people is initially puzzling ('am I actually doing something, or is this just happening?'), then increasingly engaging as the patterns of success and correction begin to register, and eventually — across sessions — accompanied by the subjective sense of calm, clarity, and cognitive availability that represents the training effect.

The Evidence Base — What the Research Actually Shows

Neurofeedback has accumulated a research literature that is considerably more substantial than most mainstream psychiatrists acknowledge, and considerably more mixed than its most enthusiastic proponents claim. An honest assessment requires distinguishing between what is well-established, what is promising but not definitive, and what remains genuinely uncertain.

What Is Well Established

Multiple randomised controlled trials and meta-analyses have demonstrated that neurofeedback produces statistically significant improvements in ADHD symptom ratings — inattention, hyperactivity, and impulsivity — compared to active and passive control conditions. The Cortese et al. (2016) meta-analysis of randomised trials found significant effects on inattention (effect size 0.61) and hyperactivity/impulsivity (0.40) when assessed by probably blinded raters — an important methodological qualifier that distinguishes effects not attributable to expectation alone. The Micoulaud-Franchi et al. (2014) meta-analysis found effect sizes of 0.96 for inattention and 0.89 for hyperactivity in studies across 40 trials.

The Gevensleben et al. (2009) randomised controlled trial — one of the most methodologically rigorous single studies — compared neurofeedback against a computerised attention training control and found significant improvements on multiple ADHD rating scales and on neurophysiological measures. Follow-up assessments at six months found that the improvements had been maintained — and in some domains, slightly extended — without continued training. This durability of effect is the feature that most clearly distinguishes neurofeedback from medication, and it recurs consistently across the literature.

Arns et al. (2009), in a meta-analysis of 15 studies, found neurofeedback effect sizes comparable to those of stimulant medication for inattention (0.81 vs 0.84) and impulsivity (0.69 vs 0.67). A 2013 comparison by the same group found that neurofeedback produced equivalent improvements to methylphenidate on parent-rated ADHD symptoms, with the critical advantage that neurofeedback improvements persisted at six-month follow-up without continued treatment — while medication benefits returned to baseline after discontinuation.

The Specificity Question

The most contentious question in the neurofeedback literature is whether effects are specific to the neurophysiological training or reflect non-specific therapeutic factors — the attention of a skilled practitioner, the ritual of regular sessions, expectation of improvement. Several well-designed studies have used sham neurofeedback controls — procedures identical in appearance to real neurofeedback but not providing contingent feedback based on the individual's actual EEG — to address this.

The results are mixed and genuinely contested. Some studies find significant differences between real and sham conditions; others find smaller or non-significant differences. The honest interpretation is that neurofeedback's effects are at least partly attributable to specific neurophysiological training, but that protocol appropriateness, practitioner skill, and — critically — the match between the protocol and the individual's EEG phenotype all substantially moderate the magnitude of specific versus non-specific effects.

QEEG-guided neurofeedback — where the protocol is tailored to the individual's brain pattern — consistently outperforms the behaviourally guided generic protocols used in many research studies. The inclusion of individuals with diverse EEG phenotypes in a trial studying a single protocol inevitably dilutes the apparent effect, because the protocol is appropriate for some participants and entirely inappropriate for others. The research asks 'does this one protocol help the heterogeneous ADHD population?' The clinical question should be: 'does the right protocol, matched to the right brain, produce specific and lasting effects?' The answer to that second question, from the available evidence, is yes.

Neuroimaging Confirmation

Beyond symptom ratings, several studies have demonstrated objective neurophysiological and neuroimaging changes following neurofeedback that confirm the training effect is real and not merely behavioural. Van Dongen-Boomsma et al. (2013) found increases in grey matter volume in the anterior cingulate cortex following neurofeedback training in children with ADHD. Lévesque et al. (2006) used fMRI to demonstrate normalisation of prefrontal and striatal activation patterns after neurofeedback, with treated children showing activation patterns more similar to typically developing controls. Beauregard and Lévesque (2006) found neurofeedback-associated changes in neural substrates of selective attention in ADHD.

QEEG studies have documented the specific frequency-band changes that successful neurofeedback produces — reduction in elevated theta in Classic ADHD, reduction in diffuse high-beta in Ring of Fire, normalisation of frontal alpha asymmetry in Limbic ADHD — confirming that training is producing its intended neurophysiological effect and providing an objective index of treatment progress that symptom ratings cannot.

How QEEG Changes Everything About Protocol Design

The single most important distinction in neurofeedback practice is between behaviourally guided and QEEG-guided approaches. In behaviourally guided neurofeedback, the protocol is selected based on DSM diagnosis — someone with ADHD receives theta/beta training because that is the standard protocol. In QEEG-guided neurofeedback, the protocol is selected based on the individual's specific brain electrical profile — and the standard theta/beta protocol is only applied to individuals whose QEEG actually shows elevated theta and reduced beta.

As established in Part Two, not all ADHD presentations involve elevated theta. A person with Ring of Fire ADHD whose QEEG shows diffuse elevated high-beta, given a standard theta/beta training protocol that suppresses theta and enhances beta, will receive training that pushes their already-overactivated cortex further toward overactivation. The result is not improvement. It is predictable symptom exacerbation — increased anxiety, increased sensory sensitivity, worsened emotional volatility. This outcome occurs. It is not neurofeedback failing. It is the wrong neurofeedback being applied without the information needed to know it was wrong.

Johnstone, Gunkelman, and Lunt's (2005) clinical database work established that QEEG-guided protocol design produces significantly superior clinical outcomes compared to behaviourally guided approaches. Wright and Gunkelman (1998) documented a doubling of clinical success rate when QEEG guided the intervention compared to clinical presentation alone. This is the scientific rationale for why BCIA accreditation with specific QEEG competency is the appropriate qualification standard — and why the credential matters clinically, not merely professionally.

The Training Process — What to Expect

Assessment First

Every course of QEEG-guided neurofeedback should begin with a comprehensive QEEG assessment — a full recording with eyes open and eyes closed, sometimes including a cognitive task condition, compared against a normative database. The QEEG identifies the individual's specific EEG phenotype, determines the frequency-band targets for training, identifies coherence abnormalities that need addressing, and establishes the baseline against which progress will be measured. Without this baseline, there is no rational basis for protocol selection and no objective means of monitoring training effects.

The QEEG assessment is typically repeated at intervals during training — every 10–15 sessions or whenever the clinical picture suggests significant change — to document progress and adjust protocols as the brain reorganises. As training proceeds and patterns shift, the initial protocol may become less appropriate. Theta that was elevated in session one may have normalised by session fifteen; continuing to train theta suppression when it is no longer elevated is counterproductive. QEEG-guided adjustment is what separates skilled practice from mechanical template application.

How Many Sessions — Realistic Expectations

The research literature consistently identifies 40 sessions as the minimum course for most ADHD presentations to produce durable neurophysiological change — not necessarily symptom reduction (which may appear earlier), but the neuroplastic consolidation that allows changes to persist after training stops. Some individuals require fewer sessions; complex presentations, significant comorbidities, or more severe baseline dysregulation typically require 60–80 sessions.

Sessions are optimally conducted 2–3 times per week. This spacing allows each session's changes to begin integrating neurophysiologically before the next session adds another layer. Daily neurofeedback may accelerate initial changes but can overwhelm the brain's integrative capacity. Weekly sessions are common in practice because of scheduling convenience but are suboptimal for neuroplastic consolidation — the brain needs reinforcement frequently enough that new patterns are consolidated before drifting back.

The trajectory of improvement is rarely linear. Most individuals notice modest changes in the first 10–15 sessions — sleep improving, emotional reactivity slightly reduced, a quality of mental quiet that may feel unfamiliar. Between sessions 15 and 30, more substantial changes typically emerge: sustained attention improving, impulsivity reducing, hyperfocus becoming more controllable. By session 40, changes have usually consolidated to a degree apparent to others as well as to the individual. Not everyone follows this trajectory; some show faster response, some slower, and some require protocol adjustment when progress plateaus.

The Temporary Worsening Phenomenon

It is important to prepare individuals — and parents of children undertaking neurofeedback — for the possibility of temporary symptom worsening in the first few sessions, and at intervals when significant protocol shifts occur. This reflects the brain's initial resistance to changing patterns established over years. The arousal associated with the first few sessions of Ring of Fire downtraining protocol may temporarily increase the cortical excitability it is ultimately aiming to reduce, before the inhibitory training takes hold. The theta suppression of Classic ADHD protocol may initially increase the feeling of cognitive effort before the brain learns to sustain beta-range activity spontaneously.

A practitioner who has not prepared the individual for this possibility risks losing them from training at precisely the point where the brain is beginning to change — when persistence is most important. A practitioner who encounters worsening and does not adjust the protocol in response is applying the same training regardless of the brain's feedback. QEEG monitoring makes the distinction between productive adjustment and counterproductive perseverance.

Home Neurofeedback — Accessible but Limited

Consumer neurofeedback devices — Muse, Neurosity, Emotiv, BrainLink, and others — have made some form of EEG-based feedback accessible outside specialist clinics. For some individuals they provide a useful complement to formal training or a way of maintaining training effects after a clinical course has completed.

Their limitations relative to clinical neurofeedback are significant. Consumer devices typically use fewer electrodes (1–8 versus 19–128 in clinical systems), providing substantially less spatial resolution. They do not compare against normative databases. They apply generic protocols without assessment of the individual's specific neurophysiological profile. For individuals with Ring of Fire ADHD, an incorrectly applied home protocol targeting the wrong frequency band could worsen their presentation — a risk that clinical QEEG assessment eliminates.

The appropriate role of consumer neurofeedback is as a complement, not a replacement: potentially valuable for maintaining effects between or after clinical sessions, for individuals whose training targets are well-established, under the guidance of a practitioner who has established the appropriate protocol through QEEG assessment. Using a consumer device without professional QEEG assessment as a first-line approach is not recommended for the same reason that self-prescribing medication without a diagnosis would not be.

Neurofeedback Compared to Medication — An Honest Comparison

Stimulant medication produces larger short-term effects on ADHD symptoms than neurofeedback. Within days to weeks, medication typically produces more dramatic and more predictable symptom reduction than neurofeedback produces in its early sessions. For individuals in acute difficulty — a child at risk of school exclusion, an adult facing job loss — the speed of medication response is a genuine clinical advantage that neurofeedback cannot match.

Neurofeedback produces effects that are smaller in the short term but more durable in the long term. The defining distinction is that neurofeedback effects persist after training stops, while medication effects end when medication ends. For an individual who will manage ADHD across a lifetime, this is not a minor difference. The Arns et al. (2013) comparison — comparable effects to methylphenidate on symptom ratings, neurofeedback effects maintained at six-month follow-up while medication effects were not — encapsulates the distinction clearly.

Neurofeedback does not carry medication's side-effect profile: no appetite suppression, no sleep disruption (typically the reverse), no cardiovascular effects, no pharmacodynamic tolerance, no Schedule II classification, no dependence risk. These are not minor considerations for a treatment spanning years. The optimal approach for most individuals with ADHD is not a choice between medication and neurofeedback but an integration of both when indicated, alongside the nutritional, lifestyle, and sleep foundations established in the preceding chapters. Some individuals respond well to neurofeedback alone after those foundations are in place. Some benefit from medication during the period when neurofeedback is still building its effects, then find medication can be reduced or discontinued as neurofeedback consolidates. The sequencing is a clinical decision made with a practitioner familiar with both modalities.

Neurofeedback Across the Subtypes — A Practical Summary

Classic ADHD: Theta suppression, beta/SMR enhancement at frontal-central sites (Fz, Cz). The most established protocol with the largest research evidence base. Stimulant medication and neurofeedback are complementary.

Inattentive ADHD: Frontal alpha suppression — training desynchronisation of the alpha idling rhythm during cognitive engagement. Slowed alpha peak frequency variant requires APF upshift protocols. Less stimulant-responsive than Classic; neurofeedback is frequently the primary intervention.

Overfocused ADHD: High-beta/gamma downtraining at frontal midline and anterior cingulate sites, with alpha enhancement for cognitive flexibility. Opposite direction to Classic ADHD — QEEG is essential to avoid misapplication.

Temporal Lobe ADHD: Temporal slow-wave reduction, beta/SMR enhancement at temporal sites, coherence training where indicated. Monitor carefully for temporary mood lability during initial sessions.

Limbic ADHD: Frontal alpha asymmetry training — increasing left frontal relative activation. Fp1/Fp2 protocol. Antidepressant effects complement the attentional training.

Ring of Fire ADHD: High-beta/gamma downtraining across multiple cortical sites with alpha enhancement. SMR as a gentler entry point. Greatest risk of temporary symptom worsening

— most requires expert monitoring and willingness to adjust rapidly.

Anxious ADHD: Alpha enhancement at frontal sites. SMR training for inhibitory control without arousal increase. Anxiety-reduction sequenced before attention training. HRV biofeedback as complementary autonomic intervention.

Finding a Qualified Practitioner

The questions to ask when selecting a neurofeedback practitioner are straightforward and clinically important. Is the practitioner BCIA (Biofeedback Certification International Alliance) accredited in neurofeedback? This is the minimum standard of demonstrated competency. Does the practitioner offer QEEG assessment and use it to design the protocol — not apply the same theta/beta template to every ADHD presentation? Does the practitioner repeat the QEEG at intervals during training to monitor progress and adjust protocols? What is their specific experience with your ADHD subtype?

Neurofeedback is not inexpensive. In Australia, the United Kingdom, and the United States, clinical sessions with a qualified practitioner typically cost $100–$250 per session, with a 40-session course representing $4,000–$10,000. Insurance coverage varies. The cost is a genuine barrier and deserves honest acknowledgement in treatment planning. Consumer neurofeedback devices represent a lower-cost option appropriate for some individuals after a clinical QEEG assessment has established training targets — not as a starting point, but as a complement or maintenance tool.

Considered as a lifetime investment in neurophysiological function rather than a short-term treatment course, the cost-per-year of durable neurofeedback benefit compares favourably against years of medication costs, ongoing psychotherapy, and the downstream costs of inadequately treated ADHD. This framing does not make the upfront cost less real — but it provides the appropriate temporal context for a treatment whose defining advantage is that its effects last.

✦ Action Plan — Chapter Nineteen

→ Search the BCIA practitioner directory (bcia.org/find-a-practitioner) for accredited neurofeedback practitioners in your area. When contacting practitioners, ask directly: 'Do you offer QEEG-guided protocols, or do you apply standard protocols without individual neurophysiological assessment?' The answer to this question tells you most of what you need to know.

→ If you have a QEEG report, share it with any prospective neurofeedback practitioner before committing to a course. A qualified practitioner should be able to describe specifically which frequency bands will be targeted, at which electrode sites, and why — based on your individual QEEG findings.

→ Set realistic expectations before beginning: plan for 40 sessions before expecting fully consolidated change. Budget for 2–3 sessions per week where possible. Alert your practitioner at any sign of consistent temporary worsening — this is clinically important information requiring protocol review, not a reason to push through.

→ Consider neurofeedback sequencing relative to your other interventions. If you are on stimulant medication, discuss with your prescriber whether a trial of reduced dose is appropriate as neurofeedback progresses — for some individuals, the medication dose needed decreases as neurophysiological regulation improves.

→ If cost is a significant barrier, discuss with your practitioner whether a home device (Muse, Neurosity) might complement clinical sessions — using specific protocol guidance from your QEEG rather than generic programmes. This hybrid approach can extend the benefit of clinical sessions at reduced ongoing cost.

References — Chapter Nineteen

Cortese, S. et al. (2016). 'Neurofeedback for ADHD: meta-analysis of clinical and neuropsychological outcomes from randomised controlled trials.' Journal of the American Academy of Child & Adolescent Psychiatry, 55(6), 444–455.

Micoulaud-Franchi, J.A. et al. (2014). 'EEG neurofeedback treatments in children with ADHD: an updated meta-analysis of randomised controlled trials.' Frontiers in Human Neuroscience, 8, 906.

Arns, M. et al. (2009). 'Efficacy of neurofeedback treatment in ADHD: the effects on inattention, impulsivity and hyperactivity: a meta-analysis.' Clinical EEG and Neuroscience, 40(3), 180–189.

Arns, M. et al. (2013). 'Evaluation of neurofeedback in ADHD: the long and winding road.' Biological Psychology, 95, 108–115.

Gevensleben, H. et al. (2009). 'Is neurofeedback an efficacious treatment for ADHD? A randomised controlled clinical trial.' Journal of Child Psychology and Psychiatry, 50(7), 780–789.

Gevensleben, H. et al. (2010). 'Distinct EEG effects related to neurofeedback training in children with ADHD: a randomized controlled trial.' International Journal of Psychophysiology, 74(2), 149–157.

Vollebregt, M.A. et al. (2014). 'Does EEG-neurofeedback improve neurocognitive functioning in children with ADHD?' Journal of Child Psychology and Psychiatry, 55(5), 460–472.

Gelade, K. et al. (2018). 'Neuro- and biofeedback in ADHD: a randomised clinical trial of six-month follow-up.' European Child & Adolescent Psychiatry, 27(11), 1443–1454.

Johnstone, J., Gunkelman, J. & Lunt, J. (2005). 'Clinical database development: characterization of EEG phenotypes.' Clinical EEG and Neuroscience, 36(2), 99–107.

Lévesque, J. et al. (2006). 'Effect of neurofeedback training on the neural substrates of selective attention in children with ADHD.' Neuroscience Letters, 394(3), 216–221.

van Dongen-Boomsma, M. et al. (2013). 'A randomised placebo-controlled trial of EEG neurofeedback in children with ADHD.' Journal of Clinical Psychiatry, 74(8), 821–827.

Beauregard, M. & Lévesque, J. (2006). 'Functional magnetic resonance imaging investigation of the effects of neurofeedback training on the neural bases of selective attention in ADHD.' Applied Psychophysiology and Biofeedback, 31(1), 3–20.

Lubar, J.F. & Shouse, M.N. (1976). 'EEG and behavioral changes in a hyperkinetic child concurrent with training of the sensorimotor rhythm (SMR).' Biofeedback and Self-Regulation, 1(3), 293–306.

Monastra, V.J. et al. (2005). 'Electroencephalographic biofeedback in the treatment of ADHD.' Applied Psychophysiology and Biofeedback, 30(2), 95–114.

Ros, T. et al. (2014). 'Consensus on the reporting and experimental design of clinical and cognitive-behavioural neurofeedback studies.' Brain Topography, 27(1), 74–87.

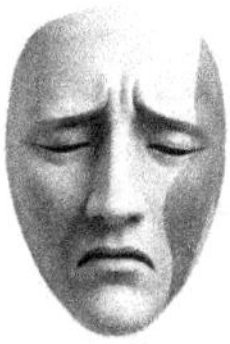

Chapter Twenty

The Oestrogen Factor

Women's hormones, ADHD across the female lifespan, and why nobody told you it would get worse at perimenopause

> ***MAYA — Age 38:*** *She has always noticed that her focus is better in the first two weeks of her cycle. She assumed this was a coincidence. Her gynaecologist told her it was 'probably psychological.' Her psychiatrist, when she mentioned it, said ADHD symptoms don't vary with the menstrual cycle. Both were wrong. The relationship between oestrogen and dopamine in the prefrontal cortex is one of the most clinically important and most consistently overlooked aspects of ADHD in women. Maya has been managing her hormones and her brain in complete ignorance of how they interact, for her entire adult life.*

The oestrogen-ADHD relationship is, in the opinion of growing numbers of researchers and clinicians, one of the most consequential blind spots in psychiatric care. It explains why women with ADHD who appeared relatively compensated in their twenties find themselves increasingly struggling in their thirties and forties. It explains why ADHD diagnoses in midlife women have been rising steeply — not because more women are developing ADHD, but because hormonal changes are unmasking neurological vulnerabilities that were always present. It explains why antidepressants prescribed for perimenopausal depression so often leave women with unaddressed cognitive symptoms. And it explains why Priya, Maya, and millions of women like them deserve a clinical conversation that most of them will never receive in a standard psychiatric appointment.

Oestrogen, Dopamine, and the Prefrontal Cortex

Oestrogen is not merely a reproductive hormone. It is a neuromodulator with profound effects on the brain — effects that are particularly pronounced in the prefrontal cortex and the dopaminergic pathways that govern executive function, attention, and impulse control.

Oestrogen increases dopamine release in the prefrontal cortex, upregulates dopamine receptor expression, and inhibits the dopamine transporter — essentially mimicking several of the mechanisms through which stimulant medications exert their therapeutic effects. When oestrogen levels are high, prefrontal dopaminergic function is enhanced. When they fall — whether cyclically during the luteal phase of the menstrual cycle, abruptly in the postnatal period, or progressively in perimenopause — prefrontal dopaminergic function is diminished, and the cognitive and attentional symptoms that this supports become more prominent. The picture is further complicated by the role of progesterone, which rises in the luteal phase independently of oestrogen's decline. Progesterone actively reduces dopamine receptor sensitivity — meaning that even before oestrogen has fallen substantially, rising progesterone is already blunting the brain's dopaminergic response. For women with ADHD, whose prefrontal dopaminergic function is already on the lower end of the spectrum, this creates a compounding effect in the second half of the cycle: reduced oestrogen withdrawing its dopaminergic support at precisely the same time as rising progesterone is reducing the sensitivity of the receptors that remain The ADHD they could manage with considerable effort during the high-oestrogen phase of their cycle may become unmanageable in the low-oestrogen, high progesterone phase. The ADHD they compensated through their twenties may become clinically apparent as oestrogenic support diminishes in perimenopause. It also explains a clinically important and frequently reported phenomenon — that stimulant medications feel less effective in the luteal phase — not because the dose has changed but because the neurochemical environment in which that dose is operating has shifted substantially (Osianlis et al., 2025; Saberski et al., 2026).

ADHD Across the Menstrual Cycle

The menstrual cycle imposes a predictable pattern of oestrogenic fluctuation across approximately four weeks. Oestrogen rises through the follicular phase (days 1–14), peaks around ovulation, then falls through the luteal phase (days 15–28) before menstruating. Progesterone rises in the luteal phase and then also falls before menstruation.

Women with ADHD consistently report that their symptoms are most manageable in the follicular phase — when oestrogen is rising and prefrontal dopaminergic support is greatest — and most severe in the late luteal phase, in the days before menstruation when both oestrogen and progesterone have fallen to their nadir. Focus is harder. Emotional regulation is more effortful. Impulsivity is greater. Working memory is more impaired. The medication that worked adequately two weeks ago may feel less effective.

The late luteal phase ADHD worsening overlaps substantially with premenstrual dysphoric disorder (PMDD) — a condition characterised by severe mood, anxiety, and cognitive disturbance in the late luteal phase that resolves with menstruation. PMDD and ADHD co-occur at rates significantly above chance, share neurobiological underpinnings in serotonin and dopamine sensitivity, and interact in ways that multiply the functional impact of both. A woman with ADHD and PMDD has her most neurologically compromised days precisely when her emotional regulation, attentional control, and executive function are most taxed — a combination that can produce the severe episodic impairment that leads to misdiagnosis as bipolar disorder.

Clinically, this has several important implications: ADHD assessment in women should, where possible, be conducted across different phases of the cycle, because a single assessment in the follicular phase may significantly underestimate symptom severity. Medication dosing may reasonably be adjusted across the cycle — with some clinicians and patients finding that a modest dose increase in the late luteal phase better reflects the changing neurological need. And PMDD-specific interventions — including luteal-phase-specific SSRI dosing, progesterone-metabolite supplements, and oestrogen-stabilising approaches — should be part of the integrated treatment plan for women with both presentations.

PMOS and ADHD — A Bidirectional Relationship

Most people know it as PCOS — polycystic ovary syndrome — a common hormonal condition affecting approximately one in eight women of reproductive age, characterised by irregular ovulation, elevated androgens, insulin resistance, and its familiar downstream effects: acne, unwanted hair growth, weight difficulties, and fertility challenges. In May 2026, a landmark international consensus published in *The Lancet* officially renamed it polyendocrine metabolic ovarian syndrome — PMOS — acknowledging what the science had long been showing: that this is not primarily an ovarian condition but a complex, multi-system hormonal and metabolic disorder whose consequences extend well beyond the reproductive system (Teede et al., 2026). For the purposes of this chapter, the renaming matters because it reframes PMOS explicitly as a neuroendocrine condition — one whose hormonal dysregulation has direct implications for brain function, dopamine signalling, and attentional regulation.

The connection between PMOS and ADHD runs in both directions. Women with PMOS show elevated rates of ADHD — driven in part by hyperandrogenism, which appears to influence dopaminergic activity and increase hyperactivity-impulsivity specifically. Studies have found that women with PMOS score significantly higher on hyperactivity-impulsivity scales than controls, though the inattentive dimension is less consistently affected — a distinction consistent with the androgenic influence on the motor-impulsivity circuits rather than the sustained attention networks (Hergüner et al., 2015; Osianlis et al., 2025). The relationship also runs the other way: women with ADHD appear to be at elevated risk of PMOS, suggesting a shared biological substrate involving insulin resistance, dopaminergic dysregulation, and neuroendocrine dysfunction. The maternal PMOS—offspring ADHD connection adds a further layer: a meta-analysis of over 1.35 million participants found that children born to mothers with PMOS were 43% more likely to develop ADHD, with the effect most pronounced in female offspring, likely through prenatal androgen exposure influencing foetal dopaminergic pathway development (Abu-Zaid et al., 2022).

The treatment implications are practical. Insulin resistance — a core feature of PMOS — independently impairs dopamine signalling and may reduce stimulant medication effectiveness, making dietary management of insulin resistance a neurological priority as much as a metabolic one. Myo-inositol (2–4 g daily), which has documented evidence for improving insulin sensitivity in PMOS, sits neatly at the intersection of PMOS management and the supplement protocols for Overfocused and Anxious ADHD subtypes. Stimulant medications remain appropriate in this context but warrant additional monitoring of cardiovascular parameters, given the elevated cardiovascular risk profile of PMOS; non-stimulant options including atomoxetine and guanfacine are lower-risk alternatives where this is a concern. Women with PMOS taking metformin long-term should be aware that metformin impairs B12 absorption — with downstream consequences for the methylation and neurotransmitter synthesis pathways discussed in Chapter Fifteen — making methylcobalamin monitoring and supplementation particularly relevant in this population.

Hormonal Contraception and Cognition

Research on hormonal contraception and cognition is mixed and often limited by methodological constraints, but several findings deserve clinical attention. Some studies have found that combined oral contraceptives reduce verbal memory and certain aspects of executive function, likely through suppression of endogenous oestrogen and the use of synthetic progestogens that vary considerably in their neurological profiles. Progestogen-only contraceptives — the 'mini-pill,' the hormonal IUD (Mirena), the implant — have different neurological profiles depending on the specific progestogen used and its androgenic versus oestrogenic properties.

Clinically, women with ADHD taking hormonal contraception may experience different symptom severity than their natural hormonal profile would predict, and changes in ADHD medication effectiveness after starting or stopping hormonal contraception may reflect hormonal neurological effects rather than changes in ADHD itself. Women who report cognitive deterioration after starting hormonal contraception deserve to have the connection taken seriously rather than dismissed as coincidental. Non-hormonal contraceptive options — copper IUD, barrier methods — preserve the natural hormonal cycle and its neurological effects, which for some women with ADHD may be preferable.

There is no clinical consensus on hormonal contraceptive prescribing for women with ADHD. What is clear is that the conversation between ADHD management and hormonal contraceptive choice deserves to happen — and largely does not, because psychiatrists rarely ask about hormonal contraception and gynaecologists rarely ask about ADHD.

Postnatal ADHD — The Perfect Storm

The postnatal period produces one of the most dramatic hormonal transitions in human biology. Oestrogen, which rises to approximately 100 times its non-pregnant levels during the third trimester, falls precipitously in the 24–48 hours following delivery — a drop that is steep enough to produce neurological effects in any woman, and that in women with ADHD represents the removal of a substantial neurological support that has been propping up prefrontal function throughout the pregnancy.

Postnatal ADHD emergence or worsening is clinically underrecognised and frequently confused with postnatal depression. Many women with undiagnosed ADHD find that the postnatal period — combining hormonal withdrawal, sleep deprivation, novel caregiving demands, and reduced external structure — is the first context in which their ADHD becomes unmistakably symptomatic. The inability to organise infant care routines, the forgetting of appointments and medications, the emotional volatility, the cognitive overwhelm of managing multiple simultaneous caregiving demands — all of these may represent ADHD unmasked by the perfect convergence of reduced oestrogenic support and maximal executive function demand.

The postnatal period is also the highest-risk period for first presentation of major psychiatric illness — including postnatal depression, postnatal anxiety, and postnatal psychosis. Women with ADHD are at elevated risk for postnatal depression, and the symptom overlap between ADHD, postnatal depression, and postnatal anxiety means that ADHD is frequently unrecognised in the postnatal context. Treatment of postnatal depression with SSRIs alone, without addressing the ADHD component, will produce partial rather than complete symptom resolution in women who have both.

For women already diagnosed, medication management during pregnancy requires careful individual risk-benefit assessment. Untreated ADHD in pregnancy carries real risks — impulsivity, disorganisation, and compromised self-care — and these must be weighed against the uncertainties in the teratogenicity literature. Current evidence does not establish a clear causal link between ADHD medications and major congenital malformations, though some studies have found small associations with preeclampsia, placental complications, and preterm birth. The vascular mechanism is biologically plausible: stimulants are vasoconstrictors, and vasoconstriction of uterine and placental vessels may impair placental blood flow — which has led to theoretical concerns about low birth weight and foetal growth restriction. The direct evidence for this specific outcome is not consistent across studies, but the biological rationale warrants monitoring of foetal growth in women continuing stimulant treatment during pregnancy. Notably, atomoxetine has not been associated with increased risk of placental complications in the available literature, making it a relevant consideration for women in whom medication cannot be discontinued (Cohen et al., 2017; Jiang et al., 2019). Women with mild-to-moderate ADHD who are well-compensated with non-pharmacological strategies should consider a medication-free pregnancy where feasible; those with severe ADHD whose functioning is significantly impaired without medication may reasonably continue after informed discussion with a prescriber experienced in perinatal psychiatry. This is a decision to be made between a woman and a clinician who knows her full context — not by guideline alone. ADHD medication safety in breastfeeding is a separate and important topic: most ADHD medications are compatible with breastfeeding at appropriate doses, though methylphenidate has a more established safety profile than amphetamine-based medications in the limited available literature. Women who have been managed on ADHD medication before pregnancy deserve a proactive conversation about management in the postnatal period, rather than simply being told to stop their medication indefinitely.

Perimenopause, Menopause, and the Cognitive Cliff

For many women with ADHD, perimenopause — the transitional phase of 4–10 years preceding menopause during which oestrogen levels decline progressively and variably — represents the most neurologically challenging period of their lives. Women who previously managed their ADHD with effort and compensatory strategies find that their coping capacity is suddenly and inexplicably diminished. Women who never received a diagnosis because they compensated adequately for decades present to psychiatric services for the first time with what looks like late-onset ADHD — because the oestrogenic support that previously masked their neurological vulnerability has been progressively withdrawn.

The cognitive symptoms of perimenopause — difficulty with memory, word-finding, concentration, and mental clarity — are sometimes called 'brain fog' in popular discourse, and they are experienced by the majority of perimenopausal women to some degree. In women with ADHD, these symptoms are not merely inconvenient. They are the additive neurological load of menopausal hormonal transition on a brain that was already operating close to its regulatory limits. The result is often a sudden and frightening deterioration in functioning that the woman — and her clinicians — may attribute to early dementia, depression, or burnout rather than to the intersection of ADHD and hormonal transition.

Menopausal hormone therapy (MHT, formerly called HRT) — oestrogen replacement, with or without progesterone depending on uterine status — is a treatment for menopausal symptoms with an evidence base that has been substantially rehabilitated since the initial Women's Health Initiative concerns. Transdermal oestrogen (patches, gels, spray) avoids the first-pass hepatic metabolism that produces clotting risk with oral oestrogen, and has a more favourable safety profile for most women. For women with ADHD, MHT has an additional neurological rationale: restoring the oestrogenic support of prefrontal dopaminergic function that diminished ADHD management was relying upon.

Several case series and observational studies have documented that women with ADHD who receive MHT experience improvement in cognitive and attentional symptoms alongside the standard menopausal symptom benefits — suggesting that some of what is being treated is the withdrawal of an oestrogenic neurological support rather than the ADHD per se (Epperson et al., 2015). The interaction between ADHD medication and MHT is an active clinical consideration: some women find that initiation of MHT allows reduction in stimulant dose; others find that MHT alone is sufficient without medication. These are individual responses to individual neurological profiles that require a personalised, monitored approach.

✦ Action Plan — Chapter Twenty

→ Track your symptoms across your menstrual cycle for 2–3 months using a simple daily rating (1–10) for focus, impulsivity, emotional regulation, and energy. Note cycle day alongside each rating. Bring this data to your next clinical appointment.

→ If you have a pattern of significantly worse symptoms in the 7–10 days before your period, discuss PMDD-ADHD overlap with your prescriber. Options include adjusted medication dosing in the luteal phase, progesterone metabolite support, or luteal-phase SSRI.

→ If you are perimenopausal and noticing cognitive deterioration that seems worse than your usual ADHD presentation, request a referral to a gynaecologist or menopause specialist and discuss MHT — specifically transdermal oestrogen with micronised progesterone if you have a uterus.

→ If you are in the postnatal period and experiencing new or worsened attentional, organisational, or emotional difficulties, raise ADHD as a possibility with your GP or psychiatrist. Do not assume it is 'just' postnatal depression if antidepressant treatment produces incomplete resolution.

→ If you are on hormonal contraception and have noticed cognitive changes, mood changes, or changes in ADHD medication effectiveness since starting it, note the timeline and discuss it with both your gynaecologist and your ADHD prescriber. Consider whether a non-hormonal alternative might be worth trialling.

→ Ensure omega-3 EPA (2g daily), magnesium glycinate, and B vitamins are part of your supplement routine — all have specific relevance to hormonal brain health and are supportive through hormonal transitions.

References — Chapter Twenty

Osianlis, E. et al. (2025). 'ADHD and sex hormones in females: a systematic review.' *Journal of Attention Disorders*, 29(6), 112–128.

Saberski, E. et al. (2026). 'Menstrual cycle-related hormonal fluctuations in ADHD: effect on cognitive functioning — a narrative review.' *Journal of Clinical Medicine*, 15, 121.

Teede, H. et al. (2026). 'Polyendocrine metabolic ovarian syndrome, the new name for polycystic ovary syndrome: a multistep global consensus process.' *The Lancet*, published online 12 May 2026.

Abu-Zaid, A. et al. (2022). 'Maternal polycystic ovary syndrome and the potential risk of attention-deficit/hyperactivity disorder and autism spectrum disorder in the offspring: a systematic review and meta-analysis.' *European Journal of Contraception & Reproductive Health Care*, 27(3), 253–260.

Hergüner, S., Harmancı, H. & Toy, H. (2015). 'Attention deficit-hyperactivity disorder symptoms in women with polycystic ovary syndrome.' *The International Journal of Psychiatry in Medicine*, 50(3), 317–325. doi: 10.1177/0091217415610311

Cohen, J.M. et al. (2017). 'Placental complications associated with psychostimulant use in pregnancy.' *Obstetrics & Gynecology*, 130(6), 1192–1201.

Jiang, H.Y. et al. (2019). 'Maternal and neonatal outcomes after exposure to ADHD medication during pregnancy: a systematic review and meta-analysis.' *Pharmacoepidemiology and Drug Safety*, 28(3), 288–295.

Epperson, C.N. et al. (2015). 'Hormonal fluctuations and ADHD in women.' Expert Review of Neurotherapeutics, 15(9), 1007–1021.

Quinn, P.O. & Madhoo, M. (2014). 'A review of ADHD in women and girls.' Primary Care Companion for CNS Disorders, 16(3).

Hirshberg, L.M. (2019). 'ADHD and women's reproductive health.' Advances in Psychiatric Treatment, 25(2), 112–118.

Studd, J. & Nappi, R.E. (2012). 'Reproductive depression.' Gynecological Endocrinology, 28(Suppl 1), 42–45.

Freeman, E.W. & Sondheimer, S.J. (2003). 'Premenstrual dysphoric disorder.' Current Psychiatry Reports, 5(6), 482–492.

Becker, J.B. & Hu, M. (2008). 'Sex differences in drug abuse.' Frontiers in Neuroendocrinology, 29(1), 36–47.

Nussbaum, R.L. et al. (2007). 'Genetics in medicine.' New England Journal of Medicine, review cited in hormone-gene interaction literature.

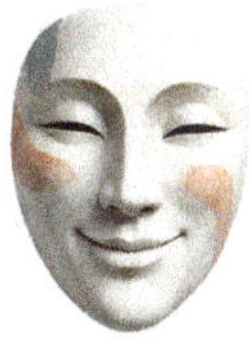

Chapter Twenty-One

A Brief Word on Work, Study, and Structure

Practical strategies — and why this is a chapter, not a book

> ***ALL SEVEN:*** *They have their QEEG results. They know their subtypes. Their nutritional gaps are being addressed. Their sleep is improving. Their treatment is being calibrated to their actual brain rather than their symptom scores. The question that remains — the one that underlies every clinical conversation once the biological foundations are in place — is a deceptively simple one: what do I actually do differently on Monday morning?*

Executive function strategies, study accommodations, workplace structures, and ADHD-specific organisational systems are the subject of an extensive and genuinely valuable professional literature — one that lies primarily in the domain of educational psychology, ADHD coaching, and specialist cognitive rehabilitation. Russell Barkley's work on executive function management, Edward Hallowell and John Ratey's decades of clinical writing, and the growing body of ADHD coaching literature provide detailed, evidence-informed guidance that would require a separate book — a long one — to do justice.

What we offer here is a framework of principles, not a complete system. The principles are derived from the neurobiological understanding developed across Parts One and Two, and are therefore subtype-sensitive in a way that generic ADHD productivity advice typically is not.

Principles Over Systems

The single most important principle for ADHD work and study strategy is this: external structure compensates for insufficient internal structure. The ADHD brain's executive function impairments are not failures of intelligence or character; they are failures of the self-regulatory architecture that generates spontaneous, internally motivated structure. External systems — calendars, timers, accountability partners, physical environment design, body-doubling — are not crutches. They are prosthetics for the executive function that the neurotypical brain provides internally.

The second principle: match the strategy to the subtype. Classic ADHD responds well to external deadlines, time pressure, and accountability structures — the urgency that the Salience Network requires to tag tasks as neurologically real. Overfocused ADHD responds better to transition protocols and cognitive flexibility training than to deadline pressure, which increases rigidity. Anxious ADHD requires the anxiety component to be addressed before productivity strategies can take hold — an anxious brain that is being pushed to perform more effectively is an anxious brain performing more anxiously, not more productively. Limbic ADHD needs motivation anchoring — connecting tasks to values and meaning rather than external pressure — before structural strategies have traction.

The third principle: start smaller than feels necessary. The ADHD tendency toward all-or-nothing thinking produces productivity systems that are comprehensively designed and abandoned within a fortnight. The system that persists is the one that is simple enough to maintain on the worst day of the week — because there will be worst days, and the system that collapses under bad conditions provides no benefit at all. Two non-negotiable daily anchors — a morning review of the day's top three priorities, and a five-minute end-of-day review — outperform a forty-seven-step To Do list implementation that requires perfect executive function to maintain.

Time management for ADHD requires special attention to the time blindness problem established in Chapter Two. External time awareness — clocks visible from the working position, the Pomodoro technique (25 minutes of work followed by 5 minutes of rest, using a visible timer), time-blocking rather than to-do lists, and analogue timers that provide a visible physical representation of time passing — compensates for the impaired internal sense of time that makes standard scheduling unreliable. Body-doubling — working in the physical or virtual presence of another person — activates the social accountability that the Salience Network responds to and reduces the isolation that exacerbates ADHD's most challenging features.

For comprehensive, subtype-specific work and study strategies, we direct the reader to the works of Russell Barkley, Edward Hallowell, Ari Tuckman, and the wealth of evidence-based ADHD coaching resources now available. The neurobiological framework established in this book should inform how those strategies are selected and adapted — and should make clear why a single generic productivity system will never be sufficient for the diversity of brain patterns that share an ADHD label.

✦ Action Plan — Chapter Twenty One

→ Choose two non-negotiable daily anchors: a 3-minute morning review (what are today's three priorities?) and a 5-minute end-of-day review (what did I do? what moves to tomorrow?). Start tomorrow. Do nothing else for the first week.

→ Place a large analogue clock in your primary work area. Time blindness improves with visible time representation. A digital display in the corner of a monitor is not sufficient.

→ Identify your two highest-leverage distraction sources at work or study. Address only these two, specifically. If it is your phone, put it in a different room during focus blocks. If it is social media, use a website blocker during work hours. Comprehensive distraction management requires addressing the top two, not theorising about all fifteen.

→ Try body-doubling for one week: work in a library, café, or virtual co-working space (Focusmate is a well-used option). Notice whether the social presence improves your ability to initiate and sustain tasks.

→ Read one of the following: 'Taking Charge of Adult ADHD' (Barkley), 'Driven to Distraction' (Hallowell & Ratey), or 'More Attention, Less Deficit' (Tuckman). These are the foundational practical resources in this space.

Conclusion

A Letter to Every Brain in This Book

> ***ALL SEVEN — And Everyone They Represent:*** *Liam has started a carpentry apprenticeship. Priya is a year into a PhD and has, for the first time, a supervisor who understands why she needs written summaries of verbal discussions. Oliver is in couples therapy with a therapist who, finally, understands the difference between defiance and dysregulation. Zara has been off stimulants for eight months and on a protocol that includes magnesium, theanine, saffron, and neurofeedback; she describes the improvement as 'being able to be in a room without it hurting.' Daniel is thriving on a non-stimulant and theanine, has taken up running, and has been in the same job for fourteen months — the longest streak of his adult life. Maya is on the right medication combination, has implemented methylfolate after her MTHFR result, has a PMDD protocol for the two weeks before her period, and has stopped apologising for her sensitivity. Amir still arrives early to appointments — but the folder is thinner now, and he no longer checks his email three times before he can start work in the morning. It is not an endpoint. It is a beginning.*

This book began with a confession: that one of its authors, using the best available clinical tools, nearly diagnosed himself with a condition he didn't have, and very nearly received a treatment that would have made his actual problem significantly worse. It is a confession about the limitations of the tools most clinicians use — not the clinicians themselves, who are largely doing their best with what the system provides — but the tools, which are blunter than we have been told, less specific than we require, and less adequate than the people they are meant to help deserve.

But the book's deeper argument has never been about what is wrong with current practice. It has been about what becomes possible when we do this differently.

What becomes possible, when we measure the brain rather than observe the behaviour, is precision. Not perfection — the brain is not a machine to be optimised to a fixed specification, and anyone who promises a cure for ADHD is selling something more appealing than it is real. But precision: the ability to match an intervention to a specific neurological profile rather than applying a generic protocol to a heterogeneous category. The ability to know whether a brain needs more dopaminergic drive or less cortical excitation, more serotonin or better methylation, temporal stabilisation or limbic de-armouring. The ability to monitor the response — not with another rating scale completed by an exhausted parent, but with the same objective measurement that identified the problem.

What becomes possible, when we add the full toolkit of integrative psychiatry to the treatment plan, is breadth. A prescription for stimulant medication is a single lever in a neurobiological system of considerable complexity. Iron supplementation for a deficient brain, omega-3 fatty acids for inflamed and insufficiently myelinated neurons, methylfolate for the methylation cycle that synthesises the neurotransmitters the medication is trying to augment, sleep architecture restoration for the brain that cannot regulate itself on six fragmented hours, gut health optimisation for the serotonin system that the gut produces and the brain depends on — these are not alternative medicine. They are basic neurophysiology. They should not be optional add-ons to a prescription. They should be the foundation on which any prescription is built.

What becomes possible, when we understand the seven subtypes rather than treating a single label, is specificity. The knowledge that Zara's overactivated cortex requires the opposite treatment to Liam's underactivated one — and that giving her what Liam needs will harm her — is not specialist knowledge. It is knowledge that every prescribing clinician should have, and that every person with ADHD should be able to access. The type of brain matters. The type of brain determines the type of treatment. Getting that wrong is not a minor clinical error. It is years of a life treated for the wrong thing while the right thing goes unaddressed.

The Future of ADHD

We are at a genuinely inflection point in the science and practice of ADHD.

The neuroimaging and QEEG literature is producing a more granular understanding of the biological heterogeneity that underlies the diagnostic label than at any previous point. The pharmacogenomics of MTHFR, COMT, and related variants is beginning to provide a molecular basis for the medication response differences that clinicians have observed empirically but struggled to predict. The gut-brain axis research is revealing bidirectional biological pathways that make the gut microbiome a legitimate neurological treatment target. The hormone research is finally beginning to document what women with ADHD have been experiencing for decades without clinical validation: that oestrogen matters, that the cycle matters, that hormonal transitions reshape the neurological landscape.

Neurofeedback is accumulating the evidence base that will, in the opinion of the authors, eventually establish it as a standard component of ADHD treatment for the majority of presentations — not because it replaces medication, but because it provides what medication cannot: lasting neurophysiological change, not symptom suppression. The technology is becoming more accessible, the evidence more rigorous, and the clinical community more familiar with its application. The trajectory is toward integration, not competition.

Artificial intelligence will not solve the diagnostic heterogeneity problem — but it will help. Machine learning applied to QEEG pattern recognition will, within years, provide clinical decision support that moves beyond the individual practitioner's ability to recognise subtypes by eye. Pharmacogenomic databases are expanding to provide increasingly precise medication selection guidance. Digital therapeutics — QEEG-guided neurofeedback delivered via consumer devices, HRV biofeedback integrated into wearables, sleep tracking systems that provide real-time circadian guidance — are making components of the integrative approach accessible to people who cannot access specialist services.

None of this will matter unless the clinical culture changes alongside the tools. The fifteen-minute assessment that produces a diagnosis and a prescription, without a brain assessment, without a functional laboratory panel, without acknowledgement of the nutritional environment, the gut, the sleep architecture, the hormonal context — this is not a consequence of ignorance. It is a consequence of a system that has not yet integrated what the science is showing. Changing that system requires clinicians who know what is possible, patients who know what to ask for, and the gradual, sometimes frustrating, but ultimately irreversible process of evidence becoming practice.

A Message to Everyone Reading This

If you have ADHD — or think you might, or are raising someone who has, or love someone who is struggling with a label that has never fully explained them — this book has been written with you as its first concern.

Not with the system. Not with the pharmaceutical industry or the academic debate or the guideline committees or the insurers. With you, and the reality that the brain you are living in deserves to be understood, measured, and treated with the same specificity that any other organ in your body would receive if it were malfunctioning.

Your brain is not broken. It is different. It is wired for a different environment than the one most contemporary institutions were designed for. It has vulnerabilities — neurological, nutritional, hormonal, architectural — that are specific to its particular pattern, and that respond to specific, targeted interventions in ways that generic approaches cannot replicate. It also has strengths — creativity, pattern recognition, intensity of engagement, the capacity for hyperfocus that produces extraordinary output when the conditions are right, the novelty-seeking that drives innovation and exploration — that the diagnostic conversation rarely acknowledges and that deserve to be part of the treatment story.

The diagnosis is a starting point. It is a door that opens access to understanding, support, and treatment. But the door is not the destination. The brain behind the door is the destination. And every brain in this book — Liam's, Priya's, Oliver's, Zara's, Daniel's,

Maya's, Amir's, and the millions of brains they represent — is worth the effort of understanding precisely, treating specifically, and supporting comprehensively.

That is what integrative, brain-based psychiatry exists to provide. That is what this book has tried to make the case for. And that, in the end, is what every person with ADHD both deserves and is entirely capable of receiving.

The brain is the most extraordinary and complex biological structure in the known universe, running on electricity and chemistry and genes and experience and sleep and nutrition and connection — and it is yours. All of it. Even the parts that have been difficult. Especially those.

References — Chapters Twenty One & Conclusion

Barkley, R.A. (2011). Taking Charge of Adult ADHD. New York: Guilford Press.

Hallowell, E.M. & Ratey, J.J. (2011). Driven to Distraction (revised ed.). New York: Anchor Books.

Tuckman, A. (2009). More Attention, Less Deficit: Success Strategies for Adults with ADHD. Plantation, FL: Specialty Press.

Brown, T.E. (2013). A New Understanding of ADHD in Children and Adults: Executive Function Impairments. New York: Routledge.

Ratey, J.J. & Hagerman, E. (2008). Spark: The Revolutionary New Science of Exercise and the Brain. New York: Little, Brown.

Johnstone, J., Gunkelman, J. & Lunt, J. (2005). 'Clinical database development: characterization of EEG phenotypes.' Clinical EEG and Neuroscience, 36(2), 99–107.

Arns, M. et al. (2013). 'Evaluation of neurofeedback in ADHD: the long and winding road.' Biological Psychology, 95, 108–115.

Amen, D.G. (2013). Healing ADD: The Breakthrough Program That Allows You to See and Heal the 7 Types of ADD (revised ed.). New York: Berkley Books.

Greenblatt, J.M. & Gottlieb, B. (2017). Finally Focused: The Breakthrough Natural Treatment Plan for ADHD. New York: Harmony Books.

Appendix 1

Abbreviations & Acronyms

A Complete Reference Guide

This document provides an alphabetical reference of all abbreviations, acronyms, and initialisms used throughout the book. Each entry includes the full form of the abbreviation and the part(s) and chapter(s) in which it appears. Where an abbreviation appears in every chapter of a part or throughout the entire book, this is noted accordingly.

Chapters are numbered continuously across the three parts of the book:

Part One — Chapters 1–5 (The Label Is Not the Brain)

Part Two — Chapters 6–13 (Seeing the Brain Behind the Label)

Part Three — Chapters 14–21 (Beyond the Prescription Pad) + Conclusion

Note: Some abbreviations (such as ADHD, EEG, and DSM) appear so frequently throughout the book that only their initial introduction and primary discussion chapters are listed.

Abbreviation	Full Form	Where Used
5-HTP	5-Hydroxytryptophan (serotonin precursor supplement)	Part 2 Ch 9, 11, 12; Part 3 Ch 18
5-MTHF	5-Methyltetrahydrofolate (active form of folate)	Part 3 Ch 15
AADPA	Australasian ADHD Professionals Association	Part 1 Ch 2, 5
ACC	Anterior Cingulate Cortex	Part 2 Ch 9, 13
ADD	Attention Deficit Disorder (pre-DSM-IV terminology)	Part 1 Ch 1, 2; Part 2 Ch 6; Part 3 Ch 14
ADHD	Attention Deficit Hyperactivity Disorder	Throughout all parts and chapters
APF	Alpha Peak Frequency	Part 2 Ch 8; Part 3 Ch 19
ASD	Autism Spectrum Disorder	Part 1 Ch 3; Part 2 Ch 9
B12	Vitamin B12 (cobalamin / methylcobalamin)	Part 2 Ch 11; Part 3 Ch 14, 15
B6	Vitamin B6 (pyridoxine / pyridoxal-5-phosphate)	Part 2 Ch 10; Part 3 Ch 18
BCIA	Biofeedback Certification International Alliance	Part 2 Ch 6–13; Part 3 Ch 19
BDNF	Brain-Derived Neurotrophic Factor	Part 3 Ch 15, 18
BPD	Borderline Personality Disorder	Part 2 Ch 11
CBT	Cognitive-Behavioural Therapy	Part 1 Ch 5; Part 3 Ch 14
CFU	Colony-Forming Units (probiotic dosing measure)	Part 3 Ch 16
CLOCK	Circadian Locomotor Output Cycles Kaput (circadian clock gene)	Part 3 Ch 17
CNS	Central Nervous System	Part 2 Ch 6; Part 3 Ch 15, 16
COMT	Catechol-O-Methyltransferase (enzyme / gene variant)	Part 3 Ch 14, 15
CPT	Continuous Performance Test	Part 2 Ch 6, 7; Part 3 Ch 14
CT	Computed Tomography (brain scan)	Part 1 Ch 4
D2	Dopamine Receptor Type 2	Part 1 Ch 4
D3	Dopamine Receptor Type 3 / Vitamin D3 (context-dependent)	Part 1 Ch 4; Part 3 Ch 15
DAT	Dopamine Transporter	Part 1 Ch 5; Part 2 Ch 7
DAT1	Dopamine Transporter Gene (SLC6A3)	Part 2 Ch 7
DHA	Docosahexaenoic Acid (omega-3 fatty acid)	Part 2 Ch 8; Part 3 Ch 15, 16
DMN	Default Mode Network	Part 1 Ch 4; Part 2 Ch 8
DNA	Deoxyribonucleic Acid	Part 1 Ch 4; Part 3 Ch 15

Abbreviation	Full Form	Where Used
DRD4	Dopamine Receptor D4 Gene	Part 2 Ch 7
DSM	Diagnostic and Statistical Manual of Mental Disorders	Part 1 Ch 1–5; Part 2 Ch 6–13
DSM-5	Diagnostic and Statistical Manual of Mental Disorders, 5th Edition	Part 1 Ch 1, 2, 3, 4, 5; Part 2 Ch 6–13
DSM-IV	Diagnostic and Statistical Manual of Mental Disorders, 4th Edition	Part 1 Ch 1, 2
DUSP6	Dual Specificity Phosphatase 6 (ADHD risk gene)	Part 1 Ch 4
EEG	Electroencephalogram / Electroencephalography	Part 1 Ch 4; Part 2 Ch 6–13; Part 3 Ch 19
ENT	Ear, Nose and Throat (specialist)	Part 3 Ch 16
EPA	Eicosapentaenoic Acid (omega-3 fatty acid)	Part 2 Ch 8, 11, 12; Part 3 Ch 15, 16, 18
FDA	Food and Drug Administration (United States)	Part 1 Ch 4
FOXP2	Forkhead Box Protein P2 (ADHD risk gene; synapse formation)	Part 1 Ch 4
GABA	Gamma-Aminobutyric Acid (inhibitory neurotransmitter)	Part 1 Ch 4; Part 2 Ch 7, 10, 12, 13; Part 3 Ch 15, 16, 18
GI	Gastrointestinal	Part 3 Ch 15, 16
GP	General Practitioner	Part 3 Ch 14, 15, 19, 20
GWAS	Genome-Wide Association Study	Part 1 Ch 2, 3, 4
HIIT	High-Intensity Interval Training	Part 3 Ch 18
HRT	Hormone Replacement Therapy (older term; now MHT)	Part 3 Ch 20
HRV	Heart Rate Variability	Part 2 Ch 13; Part 3 Ch 18, 19
IBS	Irritable Bowel Syndrome	Part 1 Ch 3; Part 3 Ch 16
IQ	Intelligence Quotient	Part 1 Ch 5; Part 2 Ch 6
IU	International Units (vitamin dosing)	Part 3 Ch 15
IUD	Intrauterine Device	Part 3 Ch 20
IVA	Integrated Visual and Auditory Continuous Performance Test	Part 2 Ch 6, 7
K2	Vitamin K2 (menaquinone-7 form, MK-7)	Part 3 Ch 15
MAO-A	Monoamine Oxidase A (dopamine-degrading enzyme)	Part 1 Ch 5
MAO-B	Monoamine Oxidase B (dopamine-degrading enzyme)	Part 1 Ch 5

Abbreviation	Full Form	Where Used
MHT	Menopausal Hormone Therapy	Part 3 Ch 20
MK-7	Menaquinone-7 (form of vitamin K2)	Part 3 Ch 15
MR	Magnetic Resonance (spectroscopy context)	Part 2 Ch 8
MRI	Magnetic Resonance Imaging	Part 1 Ch 4; Part 2 Ch 6
MTA	Multimodal Treatment Study of Children with ADHD	Part 1 Ch 5
MTHF	Methyltetrahydrofolate (active folate; see 5-MTHF)	Part 3 Ch 15
MTHFR	Methylenetetrahydrofolate Reductase (enzyme / gene variant)	Part 3 Ch 14, 15
NAC	N-Acetylcysteine	Part 2 Ch 8, 12; Part 3 Ch 18
NEBA	Neuropsychiatric EEG-Based Assessment Aid (FDA-cleared system)	Part 1 Ch 4
NET1	Noradrenaline Transporter Gene (SLC6A2)	Part 2 Ch 7
NHMRC	National Health and Medical Research Council (Australia)	Part 1 Ch 5
NICE	National Institute for Health and Care Excellence (UK)	Part 1 Ch 5
NIMH	National Institute of Mental Health (United States)	Part 1 Ch 2, 5
NMDA	N-Methyl-D-Aspartate (glutamate receptor subtype)	Part 2 Ch 9; Part 3 Ch 18
OCD	Obsessive-Compulsive Disorder	Part 2 Ch 9; Part 3 Ch 18
OPC	Oligomeric Proanthocyanidins (antioxidant supplement)	Part 3 Ch 18
P300	P300 Event-Related Potential (EEG measure of attentional allocation)	Part 1 Ch 4; Part 2 Ch 7
P5P	Pyridoxal-5-Phosphate (active form of vitamin B6)	Part 2 Ch 10; Part 3 Ch 18
PET	Positron Emission Tomography	Part 1 Ch 4, 5
PIDD1	P53-Induced Death Domain Protein 1 (ADHD epigenetic marker)	Part 1 Ch 4
PMDD	Premenstrual Dysphoric Disorder	Part 3 Ch 20
PNAS	Proceedings of the National Academy of Sciences (journal)	Part 1 Ch 4
QEEG	Quantitative Electroencephalogram / Electroencephalography	Part 1 Ch 4; Part 2 Ch 6–13; Part 3 Ch 14, 19
RAF	Royal Air Force	Part 1 Ch 1

Abbreviation	Full Form	Where Used
REM	Rapid Eye Movement (sleep stage)	Part 3 Ch 17
RLS	Restless Legs Syndrome	Part 3 Ch 17, 18
RSD	Rejection Sensitive Dysphoria	Part 1 Ch 2, 3; Part 2 Ch 11
SAMe	S-Adenosylmethionine	Part 2 Ch 8, 11; Part 3 Ch 18
SCP	Slow Cortical Potentials (neurofeedback approach)	Part 3 Ch 19
SMR	Sensorimotor Rhythm (12–15 Hz EEG frequency)	Part 2 Ch 7–13; Part 3 Ch 19
SNRI	Serotonin-Noradrenaline Reuptake Inhibitor	Part 2 Ch 13; Part 3 Ch 14, 20
SORCS3	Sortilin-Related VPS10 Domain Containing Receptor 3 (ADHD risk gene)	Part 1 Ch 4
SPECT	Single Photon Emission Computed Tomography	Part 2 Ch 6–13
SSRI	Selective Serotonin Reuptake Inhibitor	Part 2 Ch 9, 13; Part 3 Ch 14, 20
T3	Triiodothyronine (thyroid hormone)	Part 3 Ch 14
T4	Thyroxine (thyroid hormone)	Part 3 Ch 14
TBR	Theta/Beta Ratio (QEEG measure)	Part 1 Ch 4; Part 2 Ch 7, 8
TOVA	Test of Variables of Attention	Part 2 Ch 6, 7; Part 3 Ch 14
TSH	Thyroid-Stimulating Hormone	Part 3 Ch 14
UV	Ultraviolet (radiation, relevant to vitamin D synthesis)	Part 3 Ch 15
UVB	Ultraviolet B (wavelength that drives vitamin D synthesis)	Part 3 Ch 15
VNTR	Variable Number Tandem Repeat (genetic polymorphism type)	Part 2 Ch 7
WAIS	Wechsler Adult Intelligence Scale	Part 2 Ch 6
WAIS-IV	Wechsler Adult Intelligence Scale, Fourth Edition	Part 2 Ch 6
fMRI	Functional Magnetic Resonance Imaging	Part 2 Ch 6; Part 3 Ch 19

Notes on Selected Abbreviations

ADHD

Attention Deficit Hyperactivity Disorder appears on virtually every page of this book. It is introduced and defined in Part One, Chapter Two, and its biological heterogeneity is the central argument of the entire work. The abbreviation is used from the Introduction onwards without repetitive expansion.

DSM / DSM-5 / DSM-IV

The Diagnostic and Statistical Manual of Mental Disorders is produced by the American Psychiatric Association and is the primary diagnostic reference for ADHD in clinical practice. DSM-5 (fifth edition, 2013) is the current version. DSM-IV (fourth edition, 1994) is referenced historically.

QEEG

Quantitative Electroencephalography is the neurophysiological assessment tool central to the book's brain-based approach. Introduced in Part One (Chapter Four) and used extensively throughout Part Two for subtype characterisation and Part Three for treatment guidance.

MTHFR / COMT

These two gene variants are discussed in detail in Part Three, Chapter Fifteen. MTHFR (methylenetetrahydrofolate reductase) governs folate metabolism and methylation capacity. COMT (catechol-O-methyltransferase) governs dopamine clearance in the prefrontal cortex. Both have direct implications for neurotransmitter synthesis, supplement selection, and medication response.

SMR

The Sensorimotor Rhythm (12–15 Hz) is a specific EEG frequency band associated with calm, alert readiness and inhibitory motor control. SMR training is a neurofeedback protocol component relevant to multiple ADHD subtypes, particularly Classic, Temporal Lobe, Ring of Fire, and Anxious.

5-HTP

5-Hydroxytryptophan is the immediate amino acid precursor to serotonin, one step beyond L-tryptophan in the serotonin synthesis pathway. It is discussed as a supplement for Overfocused, Limbic, and Ring of Fire subtypes. It should not be combined with SSRIs or SNRIs without medical supervision.

MTA

The Multimodal Treatment Study of Children with ADHD is the largest and most influential clinical trial of ADHD treatment ever conducted. Its 14-month headline findings reshaped prescribing globally; its 36-month and 16-year follow-up data — showing disappearance of the medication advantage — are discussed in detail in Part One, Chapter Five.

BCIA

The Biofeedback Certification International Alliance is the professional body that accredits neurofeedback and biofeedback practitioners. BCIA accreditation is recommended as the minimum competency standard for clinical neurofeedback, with specific QEEG competency required for the individualised protocol design described in this book.

SPECT

Single Photon Emission Computed Tomography produces three-dimensional maps of cerebral blood flow as a proxy for brain activity. Daniel Amen's SPECT-based typology of ADHD subtypes provides significant evidential context for Part Two. SPECT is clinically valuable but involves ionising radiation and is not required for routine assessment where QEEG is available.

Appendix 2

Neurotransmitters, Brain Areas & ADHD Subtypes

Functions, Dysregulation Patterns, and Subtype-Specific Interventions

Section 1 — Neurotransmitter Functions and ADHD Subtype Implications

The table below describes each major neurotransmitter and neuromodulator relevant to ADHD: its general function, the key brain regions where it acts, which ADHD subtype(s) it is primarily implicated in, and the direction of dysregulation. Understanding these distinctions is the neurochemical foundation for the subtype-specific treatment approach developed in Parts Two and Three.

Neurotransmitter	General Function	Key Brain Areas	ADHD Subtype(s) Implicated	Direction of Dysregulation
MONOAMINES				
Dopamine (DA)	Reward prediction & motivation; effort allocation; reinforcement learning; working memory; executive function initiation; movement co-ordination	Prefrontal cortex (executive control) Ventral tegmental area → nucleus accumbens (reward) Caudate/striatum (motor & habit learning) Substantia nigra (motor)	**Classic ADHD** (primary — ↓ mesocortical DA) **Inattentive** (↓ dopaminergic drive) **Limbic** (↓ motivational DA) **Anxious** (imbalanced DA/NA ratio)	↓ Prefrontal dopamine (underactivation) ↑ Phasic DA response to novelty (hyperfocus/ impulsivity)
Noradrenaline (NA) (Norepinephrine)	Signal-to-noise optimisation in prefrontal networks; arousal regulation; alertness; stress response (fight-or-flight); attention filtering; working memory maintenance	Locus coeruleus (primary source) Prefrontal cortex (attentional filtering) Amygdala (threat/stress) Hippocampus (memory consolidation)	**Classic ADHD** (↓ prefrontal NA → poor signal filtering) **Anxious ADHD** (↑ NA → hypervigilance) **Temporal Lobe** (overactive stress response) **Limbic** (↑ threat sensitivity)	↓ Prefrontal NA in Classic/Inattentive ↑ NA in Anxious/Ring of Fire (sympathetic dominance)
Serotonin (5-HT)	Mood regulation; cognitive flexibility; behavioural inhibition; impulse control (long-loop); suppression of repetitive behaviour; satiety; sleep architecture; pain modulation	Raphe nuclei (brainstem source) Anterior cingulate cortex (conflict monitoring) Prefrontal cortex (impulse inhibition) Basal ganglia (behavioural looping) Limbic system (mood)	**Overfocused ADHD** (primary — ↓ serotonergic inhibition of ACC → cognitive looping) **Limbic ADHD** (↓ mood-regulatory serotonin) **Ring of Fire** (secondary — serotonergic anti-inflammatory role)	↓ Serotonin leads to perseveration, rigidity, and mood instability

Neurotransmitter	General Function	Key Brain Areas	ADHD Subtype(s) Implicated	Direction of Dysregulation
AMINO ACID NEUROTRANSMITTERS				
GABA (γ-Aminobutyric Acid)	Primary inhibitory neurotransmitter of the CNS; reduces neuronal excitability; suppresses excess signalling; gates sensory input; modulates anxiety; supports sleep onset and maintenance; controls seizure threshold	Widespread — all cortical regions Cerebellum (motor inhibition) Hippocampus (memory gating) Amygdala (anxiety dampening) Basal ganglia (movement suppression) Thalamus (sensory gating)	**Temporal Lobe** (primary — ↓ GABA → temporal instability / micro-seizure activity) **Ring of Fire** (primary — ↓ GABAergic inhibition → cortical overactivation) **Anxious ADHD** (↓ prefrontal-limbic GABA → ruminative anxiety) **Overfocused** (↓ ACC inhibition)	↓ GABA leads to excess cortical excitability, sensory overload, anxiety, temporal instability
Glutamate (Glu)	Primary excitatory neurotransmitter; synaptic plasticity (LTP/LTD); learning and memory encoding; cortical activation; signal amplification across networks	Widespread — all cortical and subcortical regions Hippocampus (LTP/memory) Prefrontal cortex (working memory) Amygdala (threat learning) Cortex generally	**Ring of Fire ADHD** (primary — excess glutamate → diffuse cortical overactivation) **Overfocused ADHD** (↑ ACC glutamate → looping, perseveration) **Temporal Lobe** (↑ glutamate contributes to temporal instability)	↑ Glutamate (or ↓ GABA/glutamate ratio) drives overactivation, sensory overwhelm, emotional volatility
OTHER NEUROTRANSMITTERS & NEUROMODULATORS				

Neurotransmitter	General Function	Key Brain Areas	ADHD Subtype(s) Implicated	Direction of Dysregulation
Acetylcholine (ACh)	Sustained attention and vigilance; working memory consolidation; synaptic plasticity; REM sleep regulation; autonomic nervous system (parasympathetic); muscle contraction	Nucleus basalis of Meynert (cortical arousal) Hippocampus (memory) Parietal cortex (sustained attention) Brainstem (autonomic & sleep)	**Inattentive ADHD** (↓ cholinergic tone → impaired sustained vigilance and parietal engagement) Generally implicated across subtypes where sustained attention is impaired	↓ Cholinergic tone contributes to sustained attention failure — distinct from dopaminergic inattention
Melatonin	Circadian rhythm timing signal; sleep onset induction; antioxidant; immune modulation. Communicates 'darkness' to the body. Produced in pineal gland under dopaminergic influence	Pineal gland (production) Suprachiasmatic nucleus (SCN) — master clock regulation Brain-wide melatonin receptors (MT1, MT2)	All subtypes — circadian phase delay is disproportionately prevalent across ADHD **Classic** and **Inattentive** most commonly affected due to dopaminergic-circadian interaction	Delayed secretion onset — circadian phase shifted later in ADHD across all subtypes

Neurotransmitter	General Function	Key Brain Areas	ADHD Subtype(s) Implicated	Direction of Dysregulation
Cortisol (stress hormone)	Acute stress response; glucose mobilisation; anti-inflammatory; modulates memory consolidation; regulates circadian cortisol awakening response. Chronically elevated cortisol impairs prefrontal function	Hypothalamic-pituitary-adrenal (HPA) axis Amygdala (threat trigger) Prefrontal cortex (inhibited by excess cortisol) Hippocampus (cortisol damages neurons chronically)	**Anxious ADHD** (chronically elevated NA/cortisol loop) **Limbic ADHD** (dysregulated HPA → emotional volatility) **Ring of Fire** (inflammatory cortisol cascade) All subtypes in chronic stress states	↑ Chronic cortisol → prefrontal impairment, hippocampal damage, worsened ADHD across subtypes

LTP = Long-Term Potentiation; LTD = Long-Term Depression (synaptic plasticity mechanisms). NA = Noradrenaline. DA = Dopamine. ACC = Anterior Cingulate Cortex. SCN = Suprachiasmatic Nucleus.

Section 2 — Subtype-Specific Intervention Matrix

This matrix provides a consolidated intervention reference for each of the seven ADHD neurobiological subtypes. All medications, supplements, neurofeedback protocols, lifestyle priorities, and therapy approaches are specific to the neurophysiological profile of each subtype. Interventions are not interchangeable across subtypes — particularly for neurofeedback protocols and the stimulant caution in Ring of Fire. The foundational four supplements (omega-3, magnesium glycinate, zinc, vitamin D) apply to all subtypes and precede all subtype-specific additions.

Subtype	Medications	Targeted Supplements (add to foundational four*)	Neurofeedback Protocol	Diet & Lifestyle Priority	Psychotherapy / Coaching
*** Foundational supplements for ALL subtypes: Omega-3 (EPA-dominant, ≥1g EPA/day) • Magnesium glycinate (200–400mg elemental) • Zinc glycinate (15–25mg) • Vitamin D3 + K2 (2000–5000 IU + 100–200μg MK-7)**					
Type 1 Classic ADHD (Liam)	Methylphenidate (1st line) Mixed amphetamine salts / Lisdexamfetamine Atomoxetine (if stimulant intolerant) Guanfacine / Clonidine (adjunct for impulsivity)	L-Tyrosine (500–2000mg AM) Rhodiola rosea (200–400mg) Pycnogenol / OPCs (100–200mg) Panax ginseng (200–400mg) Iron (if ferritin <30 ng/mL)	**Theta↓ + Beta/SMR↑** Sites: Fz, Cz Strongest evidence base Most predictive of stimulant response	Morning aerobic exercise (primary) Blood sugar stability (protein at every meal) Strict sleep anchor time Blue light curfew 8pm	CBT — executive function scaffolding ADHD coaching Body-doubling / accountability systems
Type 2 Inattentive ADHD (Priya)	Atomoxetine (often preferred over stimulants) Low-dose methylphenidate (if tolerated) Guanfacine (alpha-2 agonist; sustained attention) Bupropion (if mood comorbidity)	L-Tyrosine (500–1500mg AM) SAMe (400–800mg AM) Acetyl-L-Carnitine (500–2000mg) Iron / ferritin correction (critical) Vitamin D (correct to 75–125 nmol/L) N-Acetylcysteine (600mg BD)	**Alpha↓ (frontal desync)** Slowed APF variant: APF upshift protocol Sites: F3, F4, Fz Requires QEEG to distinguish from Classic	Consistent wake time (primary) Morning light exposure within 30 min of waking High-protein breakfast Fermented foods daily (gut-serotonin link)	Metacognitive therapy Written summaries of verbal instructions Structured study environments ADHD-informed educational accommodations

Subtype	Medications	Targeted Supplements (add to foundational four*)	Neurofeedback Protocol	Diet & Lifestyle Priority	Psychotherapy / Coaching
Type 3 Overfocused ADHD (Oliver)	SSRIs (serotonin-first approach) Fluvoxamine / Fluoxetine (evidence in OCD spectrum) **Stimulants used cautiously** — may worsen rigidity If stimulant needed: lowest effective dose + SSRI cover Inositol (prescription doses)	5-HTP (50–100mg PM — NOT with SSRIs) Inositol (12–18g/day in divided doses) Saffron extract (30mg BD — Crocus sativus) L-Theanine (100–200mg AM) Magnesium glycinate (400mg) Exercise (most potent serotonin modulator available)	**High-beta/ Gamma↓ at ACC Alpha↑ for flexibility** Sites: Fz, FCz, F3, F4 Opposite direction to Classic Coherence training (frontal synchrony)	Aerobic exercise daily (serotonin + flexibility) Reduce caffeine (heightens rigidity) Mindfulness — transition rituals Structured transition buffers between tasks	Acceptance & Commitment Therapy (ACT) Cognitive flexibility training Couple/family psychoeducation re: rigidity ADHD coaching for task-switching strategies
Type 4 Temporal Lobe ADHD (Daniel)	Approach with caution Anticonvulsants if temporal instability (lamotrigine, valproate, gabapentin) Atomoxetine (safer NA-only profile) **Stimulants cautiously** (lower seizure threshold) Mood stabilisers if episodic dyscontrol Mirtazapine (sleep + mood, GABAergic)	GABA (250–750mg PM — Pharma-GABA preferred) Magnesium glycinate (400mg) L-Theanine (200mg PM) P5P / Pyridoxal-5-Phosphate (25–50mg — GABA cofactor) Taurine (500–1000mg) B6 (active form P5P) Omega-3 EPA (2–3g — anti-inflammatory)	**Temporal slow-wave↓ Beta/SMR↑ at temporal sites** Sites: T3, T4, T5, T6 Coherence training: temporal-frontal Monitor for mood lability in early sessions	GABA-supporting diet (fermented foods, leafy greens) Regular sleep schedule (critical for temporal stability) Reduce alcohol (lowers temporal seizure threshold) Anti-inflammatory Mediterranean diet	Trauma-informed therapy if TBI/trauma history EMDR where relevant Scheduling tools for sequential task management Narrative therapy (processing episodic memory)

Subtype	**Medications**	**Targeted Supplements (add to foundational four*)**	**Neurofeedback Protocol**	**Diet & Lifestyle Priority**	**Psychotherapy / Coaching**
Type 5 Limbic ADHD (Maya)	SSRI + stimulant combination (address both dimensions) Bupropion (combined DA/ NA + antidepressant — well suited) SNRI (venlafaxine, duloxetine — dual action) Lithium (low-dose; mood stabilisation) Atomoxetine (NA + mood stabilising properties)	EPA-rich Omega-3 (2–3g EPA — antidepressant evidence) 5-HTP (50–100mg PM) Saffron extract (30mg BD) SAMe (400–800mg AM) L-Tyrosine (500–1000mg AM — DA motivation) Zinc glycinate (25mg — antidepressant property) Methylfolate + Methylcobalamin (if elevated homocysteine)	**Frontal Alpha asymmetry training** **Left frontal activation ↑** Sites: Fp1, Fp2, F3, F4 Alpha asymmetry index as primary metric Antidepressant-equivalent effect in responders	Omega-3-rich diet (oily fish ≥2x/week) Exercise (primary antidepressant) Rejection sensitivity journalling Hormonal cycle tracking (especially females) Social connection scaffolding	CBT for RSD and negative self-talk Dialectical Behaviour Therapy (DBT) skills Schema therapy for chronic negative patterns Group therapy — normalisation and peer validation

Subtype	Medications	Targeted Supplements (add to foundational four*)	Neurofeedback Protocol	Diet & Lifestyle Priority	Psychotherapy / Coaching
Type 6 Ring of Fire ADHD (Zarc)	**STIMULANTS — USE WITH GREAT CAUTION OR AVOID** (increase overactivation) GABAergic agents first: gabapentin, low-dose valproate **Clonidine (alpha-2 agonist)** — reduces noradrenergic overactivation, sensory hypersensitivity, lowers cortical arousal. Mechanism: activates presynaptic alpha-2 adrenoceptors → ↓ noradrenaline release → reduces CNS excitability and sympathetic drive. Use: 0.05–0.3mg, often at night. Also reduces tics and aggression in overactivated profiles. Atomoxetine (cautious — starts low) Low-dose atypical antipsychotic if psychotic features Saffron (evidence for reducing inflammatory-mood component)	Magnesium glycinate (400mg — NMDA blockade / glutamate ↓) L-Theanine (200mg BD — GABA↑, alpha↑, arousal↓) GABA (250–750mg PM) N-Acetylcysteine (600–1200mg BD — glutamate regulation) Saffron extract (30mg BD — anti-inflammatory + serotonergic) EPA Omega-3 (2–3g — anti-inflammatory) **Avoid**: high-dose tyrosine, rhodiola, ginseng (all increase arousal)	**High-beta/ Gamma↓ (cortical downtraining)** **Alpha↑ (sensory gating restoration)** SMR (12–15Hz) as entry point Sites: Multiple — Cz, Fz, Pz, temporal sites Ring pattern visible on topo map Highest risk of temporary worsening — frequent QEEG review essential	Anti-inflammatory diet (Mediterranean base) Eliminate artificial additives, preservatives Reduce refined sugars (inflammatory) Sensory environment design (lighting, noise) Digital detox (highest priority — screen stimulation catastrophic) Gentle yoga / tai chi (not HIIT initially)	Sensory-informed therapy approaches Somatic experiencing OT / sensory integration therapy Psychoeducation re: sensory processing Gradual social exposure — not immersion Environmental modification as primary intervention

Subtype	Medications	Targeted Supplements (add to foundational four*)	Neurofeedback Protocol	Diet & Lifestyle Priority	Psychotherapy / Coaching
Type 7 Anxious ADHD (Amir)	Sequential or combined approach: SSRI/SNRI (anxiety first) + low-dose stimulant or atomoxetine Atomoxetine preferred (NA-selective, documented anxiolytic) Guanfacine / Clonidine (reduce NA arousal — alpha-2 agonists) Buspirone (5-HT1A partial agonist — anxiolytic + mild DA D2 agonism) Bupropion (if prominent ADHD without severe anxiety) Benzodiazepines: short-term only, avoid as maintenance	L-Theanine (200mg — calm focus without sedation; primary) Magnesium glycinate (200–400mg) Ashwagandha KSM-66 (300–600mg BD — cortisol↓, anxiolytic) Inositol (12–18g — OCD-spectrum ruminative anxiety) Omega-3 EPA (1–2g — mood stabilisation) HRV biofeedback (autonomic regulation — not a supplement but essential) **Sequence**: anxiety first, then attention	**Alpha↑ (frontal calm alertness)** **SMR↑ at Cz (inhibitory control without arousal↑)** Anxiety-reduction sequenced BEFORE attention protocols HRV biofeedback complement Sites: Fz, Cz, Fp1/Fp2 Avoid high-arousal protocols (beta enhancement) until anxiety base is reduced	HRV biofeedback breathing (6 breaths/min resonant frequency — daily) Aerobic exercise (moderate intensity; avoid very high intensity initially) Morning routine anchor Social media detox Body scan / progressive muscle relaxation Caffeine reduction / elimination (heightens NA arousal)	CBT for anxiety (primary first-line) Mindfulness-Based Cognitive Therapy (MBCT) Acceptance-based approaches ADHD coaching after anxiety is partially reduced Psychoeducation: anxiety-ADHD interaction model Exposure therapy for avoidance patterns

BCIA accreditation with QEEG competency is required for all neurofeedback protocols. Protocols must be adapted continuously as the brain reorganises. All medication decisions require clinical assessment. Supplements are not a substitute for medical care.

A Note From the Authors

If this book has opened new questions — about your own brain, someone you care for, or the approach to ADHD care you have been receiving — we would be glad to hear from you. We write regularly on the topics covered in these pages, including QEEG, neurofeedback, integrative psychiatry, and brain-based approaches to ADHD and related conditions. Our website carries a blog, a newsletter, and information about neurofeedback training and assessment services for those who would like to explore these approaches further.

If this work resonates with you, you may also find our previous books of interest: *The Quantum Psychiatrist: From Zero to Zen Using Evidence-Based Solutions Beyond Medications and Therapy* explores the broader integrative psychiatric framework that underpins our clinical approach, and *Neurofeedback Secrets Unveiled: Your Path to Lasting Improvement in ADHD, Anxiety, Autism, Trauma and More — Naturally* offers an in-depth guide to the neurofeedback technology described in this book.

You are welcome to visit us at www.zenwavesclinic.net for further information.

About the Authors

Dr Dona Biswas MBBS, MD (Psychiatry), FRANZCP, BCN

Dr Dona Biswas is a Fellow of the Royal Australian and New Zealand College of Psychiatrists and an integrative psychiatrist with a private practice in Sydney. Her fellowship reflects a rigorous grounding in evidence-based psychiatry that has always coexisted with a clinical instinct that standard approaches were leaving too much on the table.

Over a career spanning both public and private psychiatry, Dr Biswas has developed a practice that integrates the best of conventional psychiatry with the tools that mainstream training rarely equips clinicians to use: QEEG brain mapping, neurofeedback, and the genetic, functional, and nutritional frameworks of integrative medicine. Her interest in ADHD grew directly from this integrative lens — recognising that the same diagnostic label was being applied to fundamentally different brains, and that treating them identically was not precision medicine but its opposite. Having worked with hundreds of individuals with ADHD using objective neurophysiological measures as the foundation of assessment, she has seen firsthand what becomes possible when treatment is grounded in how the brain actually functions rather than in how it behaves. Time and again, it has been the multimodal approach that has produced the outcomes that single-modality treatment could not. She brings to this book not only her integrative psychiatric expertise and her BCIA board certification in neurofeedback, but her clinical experience of what happens when nutrition, hormones, gut health, sleep, and neurophysiology are assessed and addressed alongside — or instead of — a prescription. Her first book, *The Quantum Psychiatrist: From Zero to Zen Using Evidence-Based Solutions Beyond Medications and Therapy*, explored this integrative philosophy in depth. This book extends it into one of the most complex and misunderstood conditions she encounters in clinical practice.

Dr Vivek Sharma MBBS, MD (Psychiatry), QEEG Diplomate, BCN

Dr Vivek Sharma is a psychiatrist and one of Australia's leading specialists in quantitative EEG (QEEG) and neurofeedback. His path to brain-based psychiatry began with his medical and psychiatric training at King George's Medical College in India — one of the subcontinent's most prestigious institutions — before he relocated to Australia in 2012. It was in clinical practice here that the limitations of conventional psychiatric treatment became impossible to ignore: patients with ADHD, treatment-resistant mood disorders, and complex trauma who cycled through medications and therapies without lasting relief. The question of what was actually happening in their brains — measurably, objectively, individually — drove him toward the field of neurophysiology and ultimately to his dual certification as a QEEG Diplomate through the International QEEG Certification Board (IQCB) and Board Certified in Neurofeedback through BCIA.

It is this combination — psychiatric training, deep neurophysiological knowledge, and the clinical tools to actually see and measure the brain — that forms the foundation of Dr Sharma's approach to ADHD. Over the course of his clinical career, he has analysed thousands of QEEGs from individuals with ADHD across all seven neurobiological subtypes, building an experiential database that informs this book as much as the academic literature does. The patterns described in these pages are not derived from research papers alone — they are the patterns he has seen, repeatedly and consistently, in the brains of real patients whose presentations defied conventional explanation until their neurophysiology was mapped. Rather than matching symptoms to a diagnostic category, he maps the brain's electrical activity and uses that information to design treatment that is specific to the individual's neurophysiological profile. His specialisation in Pharmaco-EEG — using QEEG brain maps to guide psychotropic medication selection — has allowed him to assist prescribing clinicians in moving beyond trial-and-error toward genuinely individualised prescribing. His clinical focus encompasses ADHD, autism spectrum disorder, sleep disorders, substance use disorders, PTSD, developmental trauma, and treatment-resistant mood and anxiety disorders. For many of his patients, neurofeedback has achieved what years of conventional treatment could not: lasting, measurable change in how their brain functions. His previous book 'Neurofeedback Secrets Unveiled' delves into this subject in depth.

Together

Dr Biswas and Dr Sharma share a conviction that has shaped every chapter of this book: that the brain is not a checklist, that ADHD is not a single condition, and that the tools to understand both already exist — they simply need to be used. Their combined expertise spans conventional psychiatry, neurophysiology, QEEG, neurofeedback, and integrative medicine, and their clinical work has consistently focused on the patients for whom standard approaches have been insufficient. This book is the distillation of what they have learned in the process of finding better answers for those patients.

About the Book

You have read the articles. You have tried the strategies. You have sat through the appointments and wondered why the answers never quite felt complete —why you still feel like the real explanation is just out of reach. What if it is? What if everything you have been told about ADHD — the diagnosis, the medication, the story about dopamine — is not wrong, exactly, but profoundly incomplete? What if the condition that has shaped your life, or the life of someone you love, is not one thing at all — but seven distinct brain patterns, each requiring a different approach, each with a different optimal path to genuine improvement?

In this groundbreaking guide, Dr Dona Biswas and Dr Vivek Sharma — psychiatrists, QEEG specialists, and board-certified neurofeedback practitioners — draw on cutting-edge brain imaging research, integrative psychiatry, and decades of clinical experience to reveal what a diagnosis alone can never tell you. Each of the seven neurobiological subtypes of ADHD is explored in depth: from the quietly drifting inattentive brain to the sensory-overloaded, treatment-resistant one that standard medications routinely make worse. For each, the authors map the underlying neuroscience, the brain imaging findings, and the specific treatment implications — across medication, nutrition, gut health, sleep, neurofeedback, and beyond. Whether you are living with ADHD, raising a child who has it, or a clinician looking for a more precise approach, *The Many Faces of ADHD* offers something the standard psychiatric appointment rarely does — a genuine answer to the question that matters most: what is actually happening in this brain, and what will actually help?